WHAT DR. STANTON'S PATIENTS SAY

"At age 60, I believed I was looking downhill. After years of being misdiagnosed and prescribed new medications that only made me sicker, I felt like I was on a never-ending cycle. I was overweight, lethargic, suffering chronic pain and depressed.

In the Spring of 2007, I began to realize my symptoms could be hormonal. While researching this possibility, I discovered Dr. Alicia Stanton through BodyLogicMD. For me this was a life changing experience. Within two weeks of my new treatment, I found relief. First my mind cleared, then the pain diminished and my energy increased.

Two years have now passed since that magical day and I feel beautiful. My energy has soared, pain is negligible and my mind is sharp. My hair shines and my skin glows. My first thought of each day is how amazing I feel."

CHRISTINE COUCH

"My second child was born fourteen years ago and that's when the migraines began. In the beginning they were very bad, usually twice a month, sometimes lasting five days—right before and during my period. I went to several doctors, telling them, "I think my hormones are out of whack." The only answer I got was medication; it was all they could offer.

I went on a crusade to heal myself. I became a complete health and exercise nut. Although I did feel better, sadly, this did not cure my migraines. My healthy lifestyle did lessen their severity and frequency, but I always got them around my period. Then, almost by accident, the missing puzzle piece appeared in my life. My husband gave me a book about bioidentical hormones. "This is it," I said; "I told you it was my hormones!"

Learning about bioidenticals completely changed my life. After reading the book, I immediately contacted Dr. Stanton and made an appointment. The care I received at her office was unlike that of any other doctor I have seen. She actually asked me what I ate and about my lifestyle. Previously, I'd never had a doctor ask me such detailed questions. As she explained the treatment, I started to feel hopeful—maybe my migraines could be cured. I thought I would cry.

We came up with a regimen of bioidentical hormones to fit my life and needs and "poof," just like that, no more migraines! Not only that, but my energy is even all day and evening. (I do not fall asleep on the couch at 7 p.m. anymore!) I experience a calmness that I never imagined I could feel. I sleep eight hours, uninterrupted, every night and when I wake up, I am energized and excited for the day. Bioidentical hormones have changed my life beyond measure.

People often comment on how good I look. I have become my old self again and it is amazing!"

KIERSTEN HEITMANN

"Both my husband and I want to thank you. I feel absolutely wonderful on my bioidentical hormones!

Before I was lucky enough to find you in March, 2007, life for me and my husband was just "OKAY." I had gained weight around my middle and hips, lacked energy, slept poorly, was tense and had lost my zest for intimacy with my husband of 46 years at the time. Prior to learning about BodyLogicMD and you,

I read as much as I could about the symptoms of menopause and how to help myself. I exercised, ate a healthy diet, but nothing gave me the results I am experiencing now. You have taught me how to care for my body and myself. The bioidentical hormones and thyroid medications you have prescribed for me have changed my life. I have energy, my weight is stable, I am sleeping well and most importantly, my husband of 48 years and I are enjoying a renewed, loving, close relationship. Using a holistic approach, you have taught me how to understand my body's needs and how to maintain a healthful diet.

I BLESS the day I found you, my healer, mentor and friend."

SHARON ROSEN

"I am a 56-year-old male from Connecticut who has always been active but in the last few years, I had gained weight and was feeling less energetic than in the past. The coach I worked with told me about the great results he had personally seen working with Dr. Stanton.

I met Dr. Stanton in 2007 and was really impressed with her questions, suggestions and the science behind bioidentical hormone therapy. While somewhat skeptical, I used the "acid test" I always use: let the results be the proof! Well, the results really did speak for themselves. In about a year of following Dr. Stanton's medical advice and hormone replacement treatment I have lost more than 20 pounds and have more energy and stamina than I have had in years. My sleep has also improved markedly, which makes life better all around.

In October 2008, I completed my first century (100-mile) bike ride. I felt better after that 100-mile ride than I did after any of my "pre-Dr. Stanton" 50-mile rides. I am sure that my added endurance has been helped by Dr. Stanton's bioidentical hormone treatment.

I can wholeheartedly recommend Dr. Stanton's bedside manner, knowledge and, most importantly, results!"

BRUCE WHIPPLE

HORMONE HARMONY

HOW TO BALANCE
Insulin, Cortisol, Thyroid, Estrogen,

Progesterone and Testosterone

TO LIVE YOUR BEST LIFE

ALICIA STANTON, M.D.
VERA TWEED

HEALTHY LIFE LIBRARY

Los Angeles, CA

www.healthylifelibrary.com

The material presented in this book is designed to be a source of information to help you make informed choices about your health. It is not intended to provide or substitute for medical diagnosis, consultation with a physician or medical treatment. It is based upon research and the personal and professional experience of the authors. If you choose to follow any of the advice or suggestions presented in the book, the authors recommend consulting your personal physician about the appropriateness of such actions. The publisher and authors are not responsible for any adverse effects or any other consequences that may result from the use of suggestions, recommendations, dietary supplements, tests or treatments discussed in the book. Any mention of trademarks or trademarked names is for information purposes only, and does not imply endorsement of the material in the book by the trademark holder or endorsement of the trademark by the publisher or authors. Mention of products or services does not imply endorsement by the publisher or authors.

© 2009 Alicia Stanton, M.D., and Vera Tweed
ISBN 978-0-9678733-9-8

Published by Healthy Life Library, Los Angeles, CA

For information about special discounts and group sales,
visit the publisher's web site at www.healthylifelibrary.com

Library of Congress Control Number 2009931470

Printed in the United States of America

Design by Donna Schmidt

CONTENTS

APPENDIX

DR. ALICIA STANTON'S STORY

It was late afternoon on a Tuesday as I started to wake up. "Holy cow, this hurts!" I thought as I opened my eyes in the recovery room. The pain was so excruciating, at first I didn't even realize that I was paralyzed from the waist down. Then I began to get my bearings and remember what was happening.

I was 32 years old, mother to 18-month-old Eric, a physician specializing in obstetrics and gynecology and a woman with my entire life in front of me. I had planned to be a doctor ever since I was a young child rescuing my dolls. I loved every aspect of my life and profession: the deliveries, the surgeries and the day-to-day interactions with my patients. From the very first day of my Ob/Gyn rotation as a third-year medical student, I was certain that this was my field. And I knew I could make a difference in the lives of my patients.

After completing my medical training, I had worked in a hospital for two years and then, just as I was opening my own practice, gave birth to Eric. I loved my family, my practice was very successful and I was living the life I had always wanted—until I started having back pain.

At first, it didn't seem like such a big deal. After all, I spent long hours standing at the operating table and was continually picking up and carrying my toddler. However, the pain eventually started interrupting my sleep. When an obstetrician actually gets a chance to sleep at night, being awakened by back pain is really annoying. With no relief in sight, I called for an opinion from my friend Renee, an orthopedic surgeon. She suggested I make an appointment.

During my exam, Renee noticed that I was missing a reflex from my left knee, had some weakness on my right side and exhibited some other abnormalities. She was very concerned but I didn't notice her reaction at the time. On her recommendation, I scheduled an appointment for an MRI.

Back then, in 1997, open MRIs didn't exist and I felt as though I was being pushed headfirst into a metal coffin. The ceiling was about eight inches above my face and even though I was listening to soothing music through headphones, I could still hear the sounds of the machine, much like someone banging on pipes with a giant wrench. The technicians kept reminding me to be still for two- or three-minute sequences.

I had been told that I would be in the machine for 25 minutes but after a while, I started keeping track of the number of sequences and realized I had been in there for at least two hours. And all of a sudden, everything connected: my symptoms, Renee's reaction and all this time in a noisy metal box. I must have a tumor.

I started to panic but managed to calm myself down and be still for the remainder of the test. As I came out of the MRI, everyone was exceptionally nice and wished me good luck; I knew from my years in medicine that this meant my condition was serious. Then, I was asked to wait for my results from the radiologist. The technician said it may take a while because they needed to make copies of the tests. Who needed copies? I didn't ask; I didn't really want an answer.

My husband was at work and my son was in daycare. Before the test, I hadn't seen any reason to disrupt their schedules and now I sat, alone, in the waiting room. Time stood still. I stared at a photo taken three weeks earlier. My little boy and I were wearing matching white turtlenecks with denim overalls and we had big smiles on our faces. Eric had big blue eyes and blonde hair and his little hands were balled into fists with excitement. As I looked at that picture of us, I wondered what the radiologist would say. In that 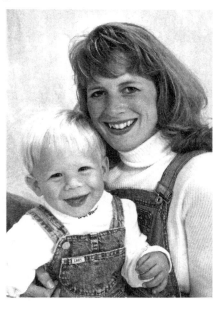 terrifying moment, I made a promise to myself that, no matter what, I would not leave my son. I was going to be around long enough to see his first big-boy haircut, attend his first soccer game, send him off to college, celebrate his wedding and delight in the birth of my first grandchild. I recalled that promise a number of times over the next few years.

After what seemed like an eternity, the radiologist appeared and escorted me to a consultation room with a few scattered chairs, a telephone and a box of tissues. I often had to call families together in rooms just like this one, to tell them that there was a crisis such as an unexpected problem with their child or a tragic loss of life. We saved these rooms for big problems—as I walked in, I was almost out of my mind with fear.

When I asked the radiologist what was going on, he simply handed me the phone and said my friend Renee, the orthopedic surgeon, was on the line. After I pushed the blinking button to connect, I heard the dreaded words: "Alicia, you have a tumor." I started crying. "Am I going to see Eric graduate from school?" She started to cry. "I don't know," she said. In another hospital, where I routinely delivered babies, a highly respected neurosurgeon was waiting to see me in the Emergency Room. Stunned, I left the radiology suite and drove myself to the hospital.

As I walked into the ER, everything seemed to be taking place in slow motion. People were talking to me all at once, getting my medical history and asking all the questions that I had asked my patients hundreds of times. It slowly dawned on me that I was the patient this time and I realized, firsthand, that patients don't have much control. My husband, Andrew, joined me as I waited for the neurosurgeon, Dr. Calgero.

As he reviewed the MRI, Dr. Calgero explained that a large section of a healthy spinal cord has an open canal through its center. My MRI showed that there was a mass taking up most of the space in that canal between my upper and lower back. Using a banana as an analogy, the spinal cord is like the peel and, in my spinal cord, the tumor was like the banana flesh. To remove the tumor, the neurosurgeon would have to cut through my spinal cord and remove the tumor inside, much like cutting into the peel of a banana to extract the fruit within. This was only one part of the bad news.

"I can't tell if the tumor is aggressively malignant or not," said

Dr. Calgero; "If it's not aggressive, you may be in good shape but if it is aggressive, there's nothing we can do—I'll stop the surgery, let you go home—you'll have a few months to live." Although his bedside manner left something to be desired, I appreciated the bluntness.

What were my odds? Given that there was erosion in the bone around the tumor and that I had experienced pain for more than three months, it seemed that the mass had been there for some time. This indicated it may not be malignant. However, the tumor spanned 5 centimeters (nearly 2 inches) and it looked disorganized, and these were bad signs. Dr. Calgero estimated that my likelihood of having an aggressive cancer was about 40 percent. So, I had a 60-percent chance of survival and that's where I focused my attention.

Dr. Calgero also explained the risks of the procedure. Since he had to cut into the spinal cord, there was a 100-percent probability of residual damage; he just didn't know to what extent. I would definitely wake up paralyzed and there was a 5-percent chance that the paralysis would be permanent. As a surgeon, I had had countless conversations like this one with my own patients. It was very disconcerting from the other side of the table. I signed my consent forms and went home; the surgery was scheduled for the following Tuesday.

The next three days were a blur as my family and I prepped our lives for inevitable change. I kept snuggling my son, who was oblivious to the cause of the crisis but sensed that something strange was happening. And I worked frantically at the office to make sure that my patients would be looked after by other physicians and that medical records were up-to-date. I kept myself busy so as not to dwell on whether or not I had a future. My mother, who would help my husband take care of our son, tried to get me to relax. My father reacted differently; he spent an entire day planting tulip bulbs in the back yard. To this day, every spring my parents' garden is awash in tulips.

I don't recall being scared on the morning of my surgery but I'm sure I was. The next thing I remember is waking up in the recovery room. My back felt like it had been beaten with a lead pipe. It hurt to breathe and I didn't have any feeling from the waist down. It's one thing to know, intellectually, that you'll wake up paralyzed—it's quite another to live through the experience.

"Good news; they weren't sure at first, but it looks benign." Dr. Nick Kulbida, my partner in my medical practice, was standing over the bed as I woke up, groggy from the anesthesia. Encouraging as his words were, the pain was almost unbearable.

Technically, no one was certain about my condition for another two days, as pieces of the tumor that had been removed were tested by two additional hospitals. In medical parlance, neurological tumors that haven't spread aren't categorized as benign but as "low grade." When the final diagnosis was given, all the tests concurred that my tumor had been low grade. In other words, it had not spread. Great news! I wasn't going to die—it wasn't even an option. When that diagnosis came, I noticed that people started to look me in the eye, which they hadn't been doing because they—unlike me—had been wondering if my life was about to end.

The bad news was that I had to learn to walk again and live with incredible pain. As I regained feeling in my legs, the pain came on with a vengeance. My spinal cord was severely damaged during surgery, as a necessary consequence of the tumor removal. The nerves that carried sensations to and from my legs were confused. Light touch caused an incredible burning. When my legs were hit with water in the shower, it felt like they were being pelted with shards of glass. I wet the bed as my bladder tried to remember how to function again.

My mother, God bless her, stayed with me for a month and helped me through the rehabilitation. Even though Eric was happy to have me around, he couldn't understand why I spent all my time lying in bed and why I couldn't pick him up. He'd snuggle up to me and I would read stories to him, but it wasn't the same. To this very day, he's very protective of me and gets very concerned if he thinks I might have a health issue. Andrew, my husband at the time, was incredibly supportive. As a cancer survivor himself, he was able to give me insight and keep my spirits up as I struggled to rebuild my life.

I learned to walk again over the course of five weeks—first with a walker, then a cane and finally, on my own. I went back to work seven weeks after my surgery.

Now, my journey truly began. I had chronic back pain, migraine headaches and residual numbness and weakness on my right side. My right foot felt like I was wearing a sock with my big toe sticking out of a hole. To this day, I have numbness down most of my right leg.

After I returned to my office and the operating room (as a surgeon), I tried to be the person I had been before the removal of my tumor, but that was impossible. I discussed the pain with my neurosurgeons. They told me that I was doing much better than expected and the only thing they could recommend was pain medication. Hospitals typically frown upon doctors performing surgery under the influence of medication, so I would have to find other ways of dealing with my pain.

I started doing my own research. Eventually, I discovered acupuncture, massage therapy and osteopathy (a branch of medicine that includes manipulation to restore correct relationships between muscles, joints and connective tissues). As a physician trained in conventional Western medicine, I hadn't been taught much about these modalities except that "there was not a lot of data to support that they worked as viable therapies," and that they might be "helpful, but not curative." My training taught me to trust surgery and medications. However, as I began to experience benefits from these less conventional types of treatments, I realized that I had held a relatively narrow view of medicine.

As I progressed, I began to learn that I needed good nutrition to support these therapies. Medical school had included a grand total of about three hours' instruction in nutrition. The take-home message was that if you ate a "balanced diet," you received adequate nutrition and that dietary supplements were a waste of money. Given my situation, I was willing to try anything to feel better so I took the advice of my therapists and started taking antioxidants and multivitamins.

To my amazement, I started to feel better and the benefits from my acupuncture, massage and osteopathy treatments increased and lasted for longer periods of time. I was able to lead a relatively normal life and gave birth to my second son, Evan, in 1999. (In comparison to the pain after my spinal surgery, labor was a breeze.) Within the next few years, I was even able to resume running, a lifelong personal passion which my doctors firmly believed was beyond my physical capability.

My interest in learning more about nutrition grew by leaps and bounds. I decided to take a course offered by the American Academy of Anti-Aging that focused on nutrition and bioidentical hormones. I didn't know much about bioidentical hormones at the time, thanks to my traditional medical education but fortunately, we have continuing education.

As I began to learn about the complex interaction between hormones and nutrition, I was hooked. It all made sense. As my scope of medical knowledge expanded, a few of my more savvy patients began asking about bioidentical hormones. Now, I was able to answer their questions intelligently and work with them to manage their hormones. These patients were amazed with the results and told their friends. Soon, more and more patients were coming to see me, specifically asking for bioidentical hormones.

At this point in my life, two things contributed to my shift into the type of medicine I practice today. First, I found that no matter how much therapy and nutritional support I received, my back would not tolerate the rigors of obstetrics and gynecology, such as standing for long hours in an operating room. On my 40th birthday, I delivered a baby for the last time. Second, I began to lose my enthusiasm for traditional medicine.

In dealing with my own physical challenges, I really started to appreciate the beauty of our basic physiology and biological processes. I realized how important it is to actively step in and stabilize the healthy function of our bodies rather than use medication to cover symptoms once things go awry.

Imagine an early American colonist being transported in time to the present day, being amazed by electricity and not wanting to return to more primitive ways of generating power. I'm like that colonist. Once I learned how to find the underlying causes of disease and prevent it, instead of masking symptoms with medications, I couldn't step back in time.

In July, 2005 I closed my Ob/Gyn office and opened a new practice that focuses on nutrition, fitness and hormone balance. That same month, I attended a conference for authors and met Vera Tweed, a writer for numerous magazines. I believe that God always puts you exactly where you're supposed to be—in my case, that was in a place where I could meet Vera. We instantly hit it off and began discussing our thoughts on nutrition and its interaction with hormones. I told her about some of the patterns I was starting to see in my patients and what I thought was happening to our population as a whole, due to our diets and stress levels. We kept in touch and talked often about the fact that we wanted to write a book together. When the time was right, we finally did. Meeting Vera has been one of the best things that has ever happened to me.

That same year, I began a Fellowship in Anti-Aging and Regenerative Medicine with Dr. Pamela Smith. I have spent hundreds of hours studying and taking courses from an amazing team of physicians and will always continue to enrich my own knowledge. I am thrilled by the fact that more and more of my colleagues are taking this type of training after realizing that there is something missing in the way they've been practicing conventional Western medicine.

I was also introduced to the incredible physicians at the Institute of Functional Medicine, who are pioneers in treating each patient as a unique and whole person and focusing on basic physiology to discover and treat the underlying causes of health conditions. Both the Fellowship and the Institute do a fantastic job at introducing doctors to this type of approach, known as functional medicine.

I experienced yet another pivotal event in 2005: meeting two brothers, Patrick and Paul Savage. Patrick is a business expert with an MBA and Paul is a physician who practices functional medicine and together, they founded BodyLogicMD. The company supports a nationwide network of anti-aging physicians with a system that enables doctors to do what they do best: focus on helping patients. That same year, my medical practice became part of the BodyLogicMD network and in 2007, I became Chief Medical Officer of the company.

I continue in my private practice outside of Hartford in Glastonbury, CT, and oversee all the other BodyLogicMD practices around the country. In addition to helping my own patients, my goal is to increase awareness of functional medicine among physicians and patients. I want more people to see the great results that are achieved when the underlying causes of health conditions are addressed, instead of symptoms being masked with medication, and when the goal of medicine is optimum health and well-being, rather than mere avoidance or management of disease. My position as Chief Medical Officer is helping me to achieve this goal.

I have the privilege of interviewing some of the finest fellowship-trained doctors in the country for inclusion in the BodyLogicMD network. I appreciate their enthusiasm, brilliance and dedication. I have also met many patients all over the country who have not been satisfied with their results from the current medical system and are now happier and healthier because of the treatment they have received from doctors who practice functional medicine.

My personal life has also experienced change. In 2006, I became divorced from the father of my children. Until I remarried nearly two years later, I was an extremely busy single mom, helping my boys with their homework and taking them to soccer practices, gymnastics classes and many other activities while running my medical practice. I also began training other physicians for the Academy of Anti-Aging Medicine, the Institute of Functional Medicine and other organizations in the United States and Europe.

It is always amazing to talk to physicians after their first day of classes in functional medicine—the mind expansion is astonishing. They have a spark and a renewed faith in making the kind of difference they envisioned before going to medical school.

In retrospect, a spinal cord tumor that could have prematurely ended my life gave me a better, more fulfilling one than I could have imagined. It took the real paralysis of my legs to help me see the paralysis of my mind. I am honored to have been a part of the lives of my patients and pray that my interventions have given them benefit. I continue to learn every day and continue to share my life with Eric, now 13, his 9-year-old brother Evan and my husband, Robert.

VERA TWEED'S
STORY

"**Y**ou saved my life," my father told me, tears welling up in his eyes. I was deeply touched but at the same time, completely taken by surprise. What had I done?

More than a decade earlier, while I was in college, my father had suffered a heart attack and on doctor's orders, took some time off after being discharged from the hospital. While puttering around the house, he discovered some nutrition books by Adelle Davis in my old bedroom and read them, cover to cover. They changed his life (and my mother's) and amazed his cardiologist, who could barely believe how healthy my father remained for the rest of his life. My father credited me with introducing him to the world of nutrition and, as a result, saving his life.

Those same books laid the foundation for my own adult eating habits and the work I have done as a writer throughout my life. Back in the 1940s, Davis began advocating whole, instead of processed foods and dietary supplements, and warning against food additives and trans fats. When I was 19, I was fortunate to be introduced to her principles by a friend in a theater workshop. I was spending long hours in dance and acting classes, not eating well, and desperately needed more energy. On my first day of following Davis' breakfast advice and taking some B vitamins, I felt like a new person, and I was hooked on nutrition.

During that era, I also studied many styles of movement, such as modern dance, mime and a variety of Asian-inspired disciplines. And since then, I've been a fan of many types of exercise, from weight training to hip hop classes.

When I started going through menopause, my lifelong eating and exercise habits turned out to be valuable assets. I never experienced hot flashes and my symptoms were, relative to most women, very mild. Through trial and error, I was able to modify my lifestyle habits to regain equilibrium.

By the time I met Dr. Alicia Stanton, my menopausal transition was over but I was acutely aware of how she could have helped me previously. I had read every book I could find about hormones and discovered some helpful material, but the sea of information—sometimes conflicting and always excruciatingly complex—left me feeling that I was on my own. As a writer, I also had the opportunity to interview many health experts, but the world of hormones still seemed poorly understood.

When I first met Dr. Stanton in the summer of 2005, I was amazed by her uncanny ability to demystify the subject, her exceptionally high capacity to care for others and her true passion for healing. Since then, those first impressions have been reinforced many times. I am honored and privileged to collaborate with her on this book and sincerely hope that it assists you in forging your own state of harmony and wellness.

1

WHAT'S HAPPENING TODAY?

"I'm not who I used to be."

"I keep gaining weight, but I'm eating less."

"I get so bitchy; my husband can't take it any more."

"I wake up exhausted, but at night I'm wired."

"I keep forgetting things, and I can't concentrate like I used to."

"Sex? Are you serious?"

"My hot flashes are driving me crazy."

*"I wake up in the middle of the night
and can't get back to sleep."*

"Am I losing my mind?"

*"My doctor says my tests are all normal,
but I know something is wrong."*

"I want my life back."

These are the sentiments of more and more women, most often in their 40s or 50s, with an increasing number experiencing similar phenomena in their 30s. Why is this happening? In our society, we are placing so many demands on our bodies that the natural functioning of our hormones is being disrupted, causing a wide range of symptoms that most physicians are ill-equipped to address—or even understand.

Routine medical tests are designed to detect disease or specific risk markers, rather than identify and rectify the problems that cause someone to fall short of optimum health. As a result, hormonal deficiencies and imbalances, even when they present debilitating symptoms, often fall below the conventional medical radar.

The whole concept of hormonal health is relatively new, and historically the medical world has been slow to make changes. In the current health-care system, change is even more difficult to bring about because business interests play a major role in determining what is considered adequate care for patients. However, a gradual evolution is under way, with an increasing number of physicians undergoing specialized training to address the hormonal problems now facing so many women and men.

Keep in mind that 100 years ago, people didn't live long enough to be concerned about hormonal imbalances. But since then, our life expectancy has doubled, and in recent years, our expectations have also changed, quite radically. Earlier generations equated getting older with winding down, doing fewer things, having less energy and zest and being forced to "take it easy."

Those days are over. We are demanding a longer life that is also a youthful one, and in many instances, we have no choice. Countless women in their 40s and 50s are multitasking as caregivers to an unprecedented degree: raising children while taking care of aging parents and—as if that weren't enough—carrying on challenging careers.

All these responsibilities add up to continual demands from different directions and hectic schedules that make it difficult for us to take care of ourselves. To say our lives are stressful would be an understatement of grand proportions. At the same time, our manner of living places additional stress on our bodies, with inadequate nutrients in our food, too many unhealthy calories, lack of physical activity and toxins in the environment. Combining all these factors creates the perfect recipe for disrupting hormonal balance.

NOT YOUR MOTHER'S MENOPAUSE

Hot flashes used to be the hallmark of "the change," and they're still a problem for most women, but they aren't usually the worst or first symptom of hormones gone awry. Initially, many women notice they have less energy or zest for life. They don't get as excited about things that should matter, or they just don't have the energy to do things they used to enjoy. One day follows another, but none of them bring much joy. They might notice themselves getting irritable or exploding for reasons that, in retrospect, seem ridiculous. At first, changes may seem temporary, especially if there has been a tragedy in the family or another stressful situation, such as a move, a business loss or a divorce. But eventually, it becomes obvious that the "temporary" cloud isn't dissipating.

Is it menopause? Not necessarily. Menopause means a woman has not had a menstrual period for 12 months, a sign that her ovaries have ceased to produce eggs and she is no longer fertile. From a traditional medical perspective, the transition into menopause, technically called perimenopause, typically produces fluctuations in hormone levels that cause hot flashes and other symptoms. In other words, conventional medicine considers that so-called menopausal symptoms are triggered because the ovaries gradually cease to produce eggs, a process accompanied by fluctuating levels of female sex hormones.

While this premise is technically correct, it is too narrow because it fails to take into account a broader context. Women today are experiencing the effects of fluctuations in multiple hormones in addition to those associated with child bearing, and most of these changes are triggered by factors outside the female reproductive organs. That's what most physicians don't understand.

THE BIGGER HORMONAL PICTURE

Hormones deliver messages from one part of the body to another, from the cells to the brain, from the brain to the glands and from the glands to the cells. This process goes on during every tiny fraction of every second we are alive. It's a complex array of functions in which hormones are designed to do different jobs and work as a team. Whether it's a debilitating feeling of having lost oneself or a bothersome lack of energy, the underlying interplay of hormones follows the same blueprint, although any malfunction is unique to each individual.

The bigger hormonal picture includes the sex hormones—estrogen, progesterone and testosterone—and three others—insulin, cortisol and thyroid hormone. These are six key hormones that work in concert, meaning a malfunction in one sets off a reaction that interferes with the function of the others.

Although nothing manmade is remotely as complex as the human body, a car manufacturing assembly line offers a reasonable analogy. The auto assembly line is continually in motion, as are all the inner workings of our bodies, including the interaction of hormones. Because the process is ongoing and complicated, a malfunction in one part, no matter how small, can very quickly cause confusion, disorder and even disaster in the workings of the whole.

Imagine an assembly line with a sudden lack of windshields and an oversupply of rear windows. All the cars are now built using two rear windows, which don't fit in the windshield spaces in the front. When the car is in motion, wind constantly blows in through gaps in the ill-fitting "windshield." The interior is impossible to keep cool in summer, and in winter, it's always freezing as rain, sleet and snow blow inside. And sometimes, the whole "windshield" falls down onto the dash, which can cause serious injuries or even an accident.

Continuing the analogy, when a woman (or a man) suffers from symptoms of hormonal malfunction, all we know is that there is an oversupply or undersupply of one or more parts, and the overall process is being upset. Which part or parts? That's where the puzzle is different for each person, and it can change over time, but an unbalanced supply essentially brings about hormonal havoc. Harmony is restored by getting all the right parts in balance, working together like a symphony with perfect pitch.

NATURE'S CYCLE

There is a natural cycle of life, which includes our ability to bear children. After puberty, estrogen, progesterone and testosterone levels increase, peaking in our 20s. Then, they start to decline, slowly at first and much more rapidly in our late 30s and 40s, reaching dramatically lower levels in our 50s and beyond. Thyroid hormone, which drives our metabolism, typically starts to decline in our 40s and sometimes earlier. These four hormones—estrogen, progesterone, testosterone and thyroid—work together to build us up, keeping bones and muscles strong and our bodies functioning well. As their levels decrease, the typical symptoms of "getting older" set in—including less sex drive, less muscle and bone mass and less zip overall.

At the same time, levels of two other hormones, insulin and cortisol, increase as we live longer, contributing to the aging process. Higher levels of insulin contribute to higher blood pressure, higher cholesterol and weight gain, especially around the abdomen, which increases inflammation. Increased levels of cortisol also contribute to weight gain, loss of bone and muscle and fatigue. And higher levels of these hormones extend the time it takes to recover from a stressful event. In short, the age-related increases in insulin and cortisol have a tearing-down effect.

Consequently, as we live longer, we face a greater challenge from nature's built-in cycle: decline in the hormones that give us strength and resilience—estrogen, progesterone, testosterone and thyroid—and increase in levels of insulin and cortisol, which contribute to the aging process. On the bright side, we have a lot of knowledge and tools to mitigate the bad effects of these changes. However, despite all our technological sophistication, today's typical lifestyles generally throw a wrench in the natural interplay of these hormones, triggering malfunctions that nature didn't envision.

LIFESTYLE HAVOC

In addition to natural shifts in hormonal patterns, what we eat and how we live influence our hormone levels and affect whether they are in a state of harmony or disruption. The combination of lifestyle factors that contribute to our well-being, or lack of it, are covered in detail in the following chapters. This is a snapshot of the elements that trigger hormonal imbalance:

- Eating the wrong foods.
- Being overweight, especially with excess fat around the abdomen.
- Living in a state of chronic stress.
- Being exposed to too many toxins in food and widely used consumer products.
- Getting too little or too much exercise, or doing the wrong type of activity.
- Lacking optimum amounts of essential nutrients.

Some type of stress is the common denominator in each of these triggers. Our bodies can react in a similar way to a cinnamon bun or an annoying friend or co-worker, and each reaction contributes to a chain reaction that upsets the healthy interplay of our hormones. As a result, the natural aging process becomes more intense, or symptoms that seem like aging start to appear earlier than we would reasonably expect. However, the proverbial glass is at least half full.

REGAINING BALANCE

We can change the way we live to reduce or remove the triggers of imbalance. While that's easier said than done, the effort is extremely rewarding and doesn't require superhuman skill or

WHAT ARE BIOIDENTICAL HORMONES?

"Bioidentical," a term coined fairly recently, literally means "identical to life." The first part of the word, "bio," means life (as in biology, the science of life). Pronounced "bio-identical," when used to describe a hormone, the word means that the hormone is exactly the same as a hormone made by our bodies. Studies that found hormone replacement therapy (HRT) increased risk for breast cancer, heart disease and stroke did not test any bioidentical hormones. Instead, they tested hormones that were structurally similar but not identical to those produced by our bodies.

To get an idea of the difference between hormones that are bioidentical and those that are not, imagine a jigsaw puzzle. In a normal puzzle, the pieces will fit if you put them in the right places. That's how bioidentical hormones work in our bodies; they fit.

Hormones used in HRT that pose health risks are like misfit jigsaw pieces. When they come out of the box, they look like legitimate parts of the puzzle, but when you find the spot where each one should belong, these misfits are not an exact match. They have extra parts jutting out, and these overlap somewhat with adjoining pieces. The spaces are covered, but the whole puzzle won't lie flat and the picture is distorted.

Treatment with hormones that aren't an exact—or bioidentical—fit in our bodies has a similar impact, with the messy or distorted jigsaw puzzle translating into health risks.

will. The right types of changes can be made in a realistic, sensible way, and that's what most of this book is about. In addition, hormone balance can be restored safely with the right type of hormone treatment. The subject has become very confusing, and news reports routinely omit information, leaving the impression that any type of hormone use is unsafe. However, research paints a different picture.

There are basically two categories of hormones that can be used in treatment: those that are identical to the hormones made by our bodies, known as bioidentical hormones, and those that are different, often referred to as conventional hormone replacement therapy (HRT). Numerous studies have shown that bioidentical hormones are safe and effective, but these research results are generally ignored by experts quoted in the media.

As an example, a French study of more than 80,000 women found that bioidentical estrogen and progesterone posed no increased risk for breast cancer while effectively relieving uncomfortable menopause symptoms. The same study found that conventional HRT, the types of hormones that are not bioidentical and have been widely prescribed and studied in the United States, increased risk for breast cancer by as much as 69 percent. Other studies have shown even greater increases in risk for breast cancer with conventional (not bioidentical) HRT.

IDENTIFYING INDIVIDUAL NEEDS

Does everyone need bioidentical hormones? No. More importantly, do you? That depends. Bioidentical hormones aren't intended to be a substitute for a healthy lifestyle. That said, some people won't be able to get relief from debilitating hormonal imbalance without using some hormones in addition to making changes in their diet, physical activity and approach to life stress. Using hormones requires seeing a physician, getting tested and receiving a prescription for your personal needs.

One or more of the following changes, described in detail in later chapters, can help to restore harmony and well-being:

- Improving your diet: CHAPTERS 2 TO 5.
- Incorporating physical activity into your life or correcting your exercise program: CHAPTERS 6 AND 8.
- More effectively managing stressful situations: CHAPTER 6.
- Reducing your exposure to toxins: CHAPTER 7.
- Using basic supplements for optimum nutrition: CHAPTER 9.
- Using additional supplements for specific situations: CHAPTER 10.
- Learning about bioidentical hormones and consulting a physician: CHAPTERS 11 AND 12.
- Putting a plan into action: CHAPTER 13.

This book is predominantly addressed to women. However, since most of us don't go through life alone, chapter 14, *Hormone Harmony for Men*, explains how both lifestyle and hormone treatment apply to men, along with a plan to get a guy started on his own road to harmony and optimum health.

Keep in mind that we have an unprecedented opportunity to live a life that is not only long but also healthy and rewarding. Life spans used to be too short for anyone to worry about hormonal imbalances. Granted, we face many challenges that didn't exist in previous decades, but we also have access to knowledge and tools to truly make the best of the rest of our lives.

2

HOW DIET TRIGGERS
HORMONAL HAVOC

*There is substantial evidence that changes
in diet are responsible, in part, for the diseases
that have emerged as dominant health problems
in industrialized countries over the past century.*

—AMERICAN JOURNAL OF CARDIOLOGY, 1972

The connection between what we eat and our health has been receiving so much publicity of late that it's easy to assume, incorrectly, that this is a new discovery. Human beings have been aware of food influencing health for thousands of years, and in the past few decades, Western medicine has accumulated plenty of evidence to support the premise. The study quoted above is just one of many, although 1972 might seem like ancient history.

The sad fact is that the impact of diet on our health, while well documented, is still largely ignored in our health-care system. Plenty of lip service is paid to a "healthy diet," but when blood pressure rises, doctors reach for prescription pads faster than they recommend healthy plates.

Hormone imbalance isn't a disease, but it can certainly lead to the development of many conditions that are classified as actual diseases, such as diabetes, osteoporosis and heart disease. And even if a patient's condition falls short of a clearly defined illness, hormonal imbalance always creates to a greater or lesser degree, a situation of dis-ease, or less than optimum health.

Like other aspects of health, our hormones are influenced by what we eat, to a greater extent than we might like to believe. It's easy to agree with the idea that a toaster pastry probably isn't going to improve your health and well-being, but it's quite another to grasp how and why that quick and easy breakfast may be contributing to an epidemic of hormonal imbalance. And, it's much more difficult to skip breakfast pastries if they're one of your staples. Understanding a bit of history can shed some light on how popular sugary foods contribute to today's hormonal problems and why you might not be feeling at the top of your game.

If you're old enough to remember the 1960s, you probably don't associate the decade with dietary trends. John F. Kennedy, the Vietnam War, campus riots and a cultural revolution dominate historical accounts, but a less dramatic development of that era may be affecting your life more than any of the well publicized events. During the 1960s, low-fat diets began to be touted as a healthy way of eating. By the 1980s, low-fat foods were being promoted widely by physicians, the government and food manufacturers as healthy options, and America jumped on a low-fat bandwagon.

The trend has had some serious, unintended consequences. Rather than encouraging people to eat more fruits, vegetables and lean protein, the low-fat craze popularized more and more processed foods with large amounts of refined carbohydrates, such as pasta, bagels, pretzels, rice cakes, low-fat cookies and other baked goods. To appeal to consumers' taste buds, makers of low-fat foods compensated for lack of fat with refined flour and sugar, triggering a host of health problems, such as obesity and diabetes.

Consider changes in breakfast, for example. Bacon and eggs became taboo, and sugary cereal, generally made with refined grains, became the "healthy" alternative. (Whole grain cereal is now gaining popularity but it still isn't always the best option—more on that later.) Although eggs are a perfectly good food that became maligned without good reason, bacon and copious amounts of butter weren't the best options. However, replacing this once traditional breakfast with sugary cereal was a case of "out of the frying pan and into the fire."

Too much saturated fat does promote disease, but the link between obesity, diabetes and refined, sugary foods has also emerged as a major dietary pitfall. While low-fat foods have grown in sales, saturated fat consumption hasn't been reduced as high-fat fast food replaced many home-cooked meals. In other words, rather than improving the American diet, the increase of low-fat foods has made it worse by increasing the amount of refined flour and sugar.

Given that we're continually exposed to news about how one food or another does a body good or bad, the more attention we pay to the latest dietary discoveries, the more confusing life can become. To make sense of the constantly growing sea of information, we have to identify the factors that have the greatest impact on hormonal balance and other aspects of health.

The most basic link between diet and hormones is this: Consuming too much refined flour and sugar disrupts hormonal balance. This fact is like the invisible elephant in the room, and it can't be overstated. Although it isn't the only aspect of diet that affects hormonal health, it is the most common factor that underlies imbalance, and its impact should never be underestimated or forgotten. To recap: Consuming too much refined flour and sugar disrupts hormonal balance.

Your reaction to this concept will depend upon how much effort you've been making to educate yourself about healthy eating, and how proactive you've been in trying to make healthy choices. If good nutrition and healthy cooking are among your passions, you may think this basic idea is a no-brainer, or you may be disappointed that it doesn't sound like a new concept. Think about it again. Yes, we've known for a long time that you won't improve your health by eating lots of sugar and refined flour but consider this: The relationship between these same types of unhealthy foods and hormonal imbalance is largely unrecognized, yet it may be the single most important dietary factor underlying hormonal havoc.

The proverbial elephant may become more visible and easier to deal with if we look at the bigger picture of how hormones interact and how food triggers a chain reaction.

MALFUNCTION #1: THE FOOD-INSULIN TRIGGER

The hormones we traditionally think of as being balanced or imbalanced—estrogen and progesterone—are influenced by other hormones. Insulin plays a critical role. Because it's not a "sex hormone," insulin is often omitted or not emphasized enough in discussions about how to balance hormones, but it is the most common trigger of imbalance.

In order for our bodies to use food as fuel for energy, the food has to be converted to blood sugar, or glucose, in our blood. Once that's done, insulin transports the glucose to muscle cells, which are supposed to take in the glucose, burn it and generate energy, like a furnace that heats a house or an engine that drives machinery. Ideally, this process functions in a way that gives us a stable, constant level of energy so that we can happily go about our business of living, but it doesn't always work that way.

> Consuming too much refined flour and sugar disrupts hormonal balance.

Different foods are converted into blood glucose at different speeds. Refined flour and sugar convert very rapidly, so when we eat them our blood gets a flood of glucose, which is why we sometimes experience a sugar rush. Insulin is then generated in the pancreas, and a lot of glucose is delivered to cells within a short time. If you were to graph blood glucose levels after you eat sugary food, you would see a spike followed by a crash. That crash is the slump in energy we experience after a sugar "high," and it leads to cravings for more sugary food.

When this spike-crash cycle repeats over and over, a problem develops. Think of it this way: Imagine that blood glucose is a pizza, insulin is the pizza delivery guy and muscle cells are a nice neighborhood of homes with hungry families waiting for their dinner to be delivered. When the pizza delivery guy rings the doorbell of a home, someone opens the door and gladly takes the pizza. Pizza gets delivered to each home and each family is fed and happy. That's how the process is supposed to work.

However, when there's an oversupply of blood glucose from

too much refined flour and sugar, a different scene develops: A home barely takes delivery of one pizza when another delivery guy comes along, followed by another and another. This happens to every home in the neighborhood. The whole neighborhood is now swarming with pizza delivery guys who are constantly ringing the doorbells. More and more of them keep coming. The families in the homes stop answering their doorbells, but they can see pizza delivery guys everywhere, in the streets, alleys and yards, so they lock their doors and windows because they just can't take it any more.

To solve the problem of being shut out, the pizza delivery guys get resourceful and find another neighborhood that's glad to accept deliveries of pizza. The doorbells of these homes are always answered, and pizza is never refused, even when it arrives in huge quantities. Why is this neighborhood so different? It's where the fat cells live. Unlike the muscle cells, which can only accept so much fuel in a given time period, the fat cells have an unlimited capacity to accept endless amounts of fuel. They may not burn it to produce energy, but they're happy to simply store limitless quantities.

To continue the pizza analogy one step further, you can think of the doors in the homes as receptors on each cell, which are supposed to respond to insulin making a delivery of glucose. Just like the homes in the muscle cell neighborhood, muscle cell receptors get overwhelmed by an overload of glucose deliveries, and they shut their "doors." When this condition develops, it's called insulin resistance. Eating too much saturated and trans fat also contributes to the development and persistence of this condition.

Insulin resistance promotes weight gain because it prompts fuel to be preferentially delivered to fat cells, and it leads to elevated levels of glucose in the blood. Both excess body fat and elevated blood glucose contribute to hormone imbalance. Insulin resistance has been receiving more and more attention in the medical community in recent years because it sets the stage for diabetes and heart disease, but its effect on other hormones is not acknowledged by most physicians.

MALFUNCTION #2: THE CORTISOL TRIGGER

The spikes and crashes of blood glucose put stress on the body which, in turn, leads to overproduction of cortisol, the "fight or flight" hormone. Stress from life situations also leads to overproduction of cortisol and is another factor that needs to be managed. However, if the insulin trigger isn't already present, the body can deal more easily with the effects of life stress since they aren't being piled on top of dietary stress.

Cortisol production is a vital part of life. As the "fight or flight" hormone, cortisol enables us to function in stressful situations. If food is scarce, cortisol converts stored protein to glucose in the blood as a backup energy generating system. Among other things, the brain requires glucose to function, and cortisol is a fail-safe mechanism to make sure our brains don't experience starvation and can continue to function, even in difficult circumstances. In a nutshell, cortisol per-

> Blood sugar spikes and crashes trigger overproduction of cortisol, the stress hormone.

forms vital functions, but like most things done to excess, too much cortisol production has some liabilities.

Normal cortisol levels are highest in the morning and taper off slowly as the day progresses, so that we are relaxed and ready for a restful sleep by bedtime. When cortisol production goes awry, levels can become low in the morning, so much so that it's hard to get out of bed. Cortisol levels can dive midafternoon, when it seems like the workday will never end. And after dinner, they can start to rise, hitting a peak around 10 p.m., so that instead of being ready for rest, we're wired and can't fall asleep. The next day we're exhausted, beginning the cycle again. These types of symptoms are well known in complementary and naturopathic healing circles where fatigue is treated, but there is another liability to cortisol malfunction that is most often overlooked. Cortisol overproduction triggers an imbalance in sex hormones because it leads to depleted levels of progesterone.

MALFUNCTION #3: THE PROGESTERONE DEFICIENCY

Hormones don't function in isolation. As long as we are alive, there is an ongoing process that includes hormones being produced from various substances and a network of interactions that is far more complex than anything in cyberspace.

Progesterone, in addition to performing certain vital functions, is also a building block for cortisol. When everything is in balance, both progesterone and cortisol do their jobs in harmony. However, when there is too much demand for cortisol, due to stress or insulin resistance, too much progesterone is used to make cortisol. The result is a depletion of progesterone.

This is where the more familiar sex hormones enter the picture. Nature requires a balance between progesterone and estrogen, and when progesterone is diverted to produce cortisol, an estrogen-progesterone imbalance is created. It's often referred to as estrogen dominance, meaning that the level of estrogen is too high in relation to progesterone, or progesterone is too low in relation to estrogen. The point is that the two are not balanced as they should be.

This imbalance is the most common one that leads many women to start experiencing what seems to be an early menopause. Symptoms such as

> **Stress disrupts balance among hormones.**

irregular or unusually heavy periods, and sometimes hot flashes, start appearing at an earlier age than we traditionally expect. Such symptoms may or may not mean that a women's ovaries are starting to wind down, but they are always an indicator of hormonal imbalance. And this imbalance may disturb the balance with other hormones, including thyroid and testosterone.

When women are beginning the transition into menopause, hormone levels will fluctuate naturally, and physical changes–which vary from woman to woman–will occur. However, an imbalance created by stress, insulin resistance and an unhealthy lifestyle will magnify true menopausal symptoms, and this is exactly what is happening to more and more women.

THE INFORMATION GAP

You might be wondering why you haven't heard more about this in the past. Medicine today tends to be divided into isolated segments and to be driven by attempts to reduce symptoms, most often with pharmaceutical treatment. It isn't all the physicians' doing but a combination of factors that make up our health-care system, including research largely funded by companies marketing medications, and protocols strongly influenced by what is covered by insurance plans. And, "news" consists of things that appear to be a quick fix, while a combination of lifestyle factors that increase or decrease the chances of hormonal imbalance don't usually make headlines.

A 10-year study of more than 28,000 French women found that eating foods which contain rapidly absorbed sugars and drinking alcohol increases the likelihood of uncomfortable symptoms associated with the transition into and through menopause.

There is plenty of science supporting how our bodies work, in medical texts that are part of every medical school curriculum. In addition, there is research demonstrating the links between diet, hormonal issues and severity of uncomfortable symptoms.

In women approaching or going through menopause, both insulin resistance and excess weight increase the odds of more uncomfortable and more intense symptoms. Given the large amounts of refined flour and sugar in our diets for the past few decades, this mechanism is a major contributor to an epidemic of hormonal imbalance. And, insulin resistance is a major reason why more and more women are starting to experience symptoms of the transition into menopause in their late 20s and 30s.

3

CULTURE AND CARBOHYDRATES

Knowing something about the insulin-hormone imbalance connection is one thing. Doing something about it by changing your eating habits is quite another. If knowledge alone led to healthier habits, the fast-food industry would be suffering instead of flourishing worldwide. And unless you've been living on another planet, even before you read the last chapter, you probably knew that refined flour and sugar aren't the healthiest food ingredients.

You've also heard that too much fat in your diet doesn't enhance health. Yet, packaged foods containing ample quantities of these types of ingredients are plentiful in supermarkets and most homes, and for most people, the idea of replacing them with more wholesome options is quite difficult to envision, let alone put into practice. So let's just agree that it's rarely easy for anyone to change familiar habits, especially those related to food.

That said, what exactly do you need to do and where do you start? It isn't just a matter of willpower. If you want to use food to balance hormones, feel better and enjoy overall health, it helps to understand the bigger picture: why certain types of foods are more popular than others, what benefits and liabilities they carry, how social pressures are involved, and the most important eating habits to develop, reinforce or ditch. Let's look at the bigger picture.

CULTURAL MESSAGES

We live in a cultural environment designed to prompt and perpetuate eating habits that disrupt hormones, injure health and reduce our lifespan. That sounds depressing, doesn't it? It certainly could be. On the other hand, taking stock of your environment can work to your advantage.

Think of it this way: By recognizing the actual challenges you face, it's possible to work out some realistic ways to overcome them. Consider some of the advertising messages we're exposed to and ask yourself if you've ever wanted to believe what they promise, if only for a fleeting moment. This is a very short list:

- Drink this soda and get a new life. Not only will things go better but hey, life will be more fun. What's more, you'll look and feel like a gorgeous 20-year-old.
- Eat this hamburger, and you'll become a stunning model (or for men, the hot guy on the cover of romance novels) who has a great life and is liked, admired and sexually desired by others.
- Eat this cookie or dessert, and you'll instantly be transported to an idyllic, tranquil place that exists only in your dreams.
- Eating "on the go," doing anything other than sitting at a table while stuffing food into your mouth, means you're living a full and exciting life.
- In a happy family, no one prepares a meal using fresh ingredients. When happy folks don't go out for fast food, they bring it home or heat up something that comes in a package.

- It's really cool to eat fast food in a car.
- There really is a pink bunny that never ceases to beat a drum.

Granted, the last one is tongue in cheek. But seriously, the next time you are on the receiving end of an advertising message, in any medium, ignore the product for a moment and think about what kind of lifestyle is being communicated. What benefit is the advertiser really offering? And more importantly, to what extent is the product likely to deliver what's promised or implied?

SOCIAL PRESSURES

If you've ever decided to make changes in how you eat, you've quite likely run into some resistance from friends, co-workers or family members. We live in a world that is accustomed to eating certain ways, and unless you socialize, work and live with the minority of people who already have healthy habits, you might as well be prepared for some type of reaction when you don't follow your usual eating routines. If you're taken off guard, it could sabotage your best intentions.

At any social gathering, there is usually at least one person who can't quite accept a polite "No, thank you," when someone declines a piece–or even a second piece–of cake. It could be the hostess or another guest. "Oh, come on, life's too short," or "Not even a little piece?" Even if you don't particularly want that piece of cake, it's quite easy to eat it anyway in these types of situations.

If you work in an office where cookies and candy are spread

around and eaten throughout the day by one and all, declining the treats might seem threatening to co-workers. You might get labeled as "the health nut," or something along those lines. And unless you live alone, other family members can have varying reactions to new eating habits.

People generally feel most comfortable with others who are like-minded. In a group, whether the connection is social or work-related, there are certain common ways of behaving that are taken for granted. If you suddenly behave differently, well, it rocks the boat, even if just a little.

Among couples and family members, changing meals that are shared requires a bit of thought. For example, if high-fat, starchy casseroles or fatty meats and rich sauces are suddenly replaced by grilled fish and steamed vegetables for dinner, the reaction may be quite dramatic, and it most likely won't be a standing ovation for the chef. At any age, people tend to be creatures of habit and are more likely to accept a gradual transition rather than an abrupt change.

Before looking at what specific dietary changes help to balance hormones, it's a good idea to be mindful of the challenge that other people's reactions might present. In some situations, other people's responses to your food choices can become a new source of stress, and stress is something you want to minimize. However, we eat a lot of food by ourselves, and a good place to start making healthier choices is for those solitary meals or snacks.

CARBOHYDRATE LIABILITIES

The most common and basic trigger of hormonal imbalance is

insulin resistance, and eating in a way that prevents or reverses the condition is a first step. In practice, that means reducing the overabundance of refined carbohydrates in our diets. While refined carbohydrates don't promote health for men or women at any age, hormonal changes associated with menopause may reduce our sensitivity to insulin. In other words, there are two strikes against us as we live longer: We are surrounded by foods that wreak havoc on hormones and our cells may become less sensitive to insulin as our reproductive hormones decline.

It's well established in the medical community that insulin resistance increases risk for heart disease, stroke, type 2 diabetes and weight gain, and that it contributes to inflammation, another factor which increases risk for the same diseases. Because of this connection, foods that help to balance hormones also decrease risk for these other diseases. And, if you're battling excess weight, the same eating habits will do double duty to help you lose weight.

There is also a link between some female cancers and carbohydrates that are rapidly absorbed, such as refined foods that are quickly converted into blood sugar. This connection is more controversial, because the results of some studies in the past did not support the premise. However, there are numerous studies of thousands of women that do, indeed, show that there is a link. Here's a look at some of the research.

- A 9-year study of more than 62,000 postmenopausal women in France found that rapidly absorbed carbohydrates were associated with higher risk for breast cancer among women who were overweight or had a large waist.

- In Italy, nearly 9,000 women were tracked for an average of approximately 11 years to examine links between diet and breast cancer. Those with the greatest risk for breast cancer ate the most rapidly absorbed carbohydrates and were not overweight in the years approaching menopause.
- In Western New York, a study of more than 3,000 women found that eating less food that rapidly increases blood-sugar levels reduced risk for breast cancer among postmenopausal women who were overweight and that higher levels of such foods increased risk among the same group of women.
- In Mexico, a study of nearly 1,900 women found that high intake of rapidly absorbed carbohydrates increased risk for breast cancer both before and after menopause, with the risk increasing further after menopause.
- In Canada, nearly 50,000 women were tracked for approximately 16 years. Those who ate more rapidly absorbed carbohydrates had increased risk for breast and endometrial cancers, and the risk for the latter was even greater among women who were also obese.
- An Italian study of nearly 2,500 women found that rapidly absorbed carbohydrates increased risk for ovarian cancer both before and after menopause.
- A study of more than 23,000 women in Iowa found that rapidly absorbed carbohydrates may increase risk for endometrial cancer in women who were not diabetic.

It's important to keep in mind that the risk factor in all these studies was rapidly absorbed carbohydrates, which are generally those made with refined flour and sugar. Researchers did not find a correlation between carbohydrates in general and risk for breast, endometrial or ovarian cancers. A link between these cancers and carbohydrates in general has been looked for, but none has been found. This makes sense, given that all vegetables, fruits and whole grains contain carbohydrates, along with an enormous number of health-promoting nutrients.

CARBOHYDRATE QUALITY

The speed with which carbohydrates are converted into blood sugar determines whether or not a given food promotes hormonal balance or imbalance, and whether the food increases or decreases risk for disease. The glycemic index (GI) is a system of measuring the conversion speed of individual foods. For stable blood sugar, the carbohydrates that are staples in our diets should be those that convert slowly, which means they have a low GI.

Keep in mind that this whole issue of GI applies only to carbohydrates. Meat, fish, seafood, eggs, cheese and fats, including butter and oils, are not assigned GI ratings because fats and proteins are absorbed slowly and don't affect blood-sugar levels. However, quantity and quality of fats also affect our health, so just because a high-fat food has a low-GI rating doesn't mean it should be eaten mindlessly. For now, let's keep looking at carbohydrates, as these really are the biggest category of culprits in our health, not because all carbohydrates are inherently bad but because our culture heavily promotes the ones that do damage.

In the simplest terms, if you ate only non-starchy vegetables and lean proteins, with some fresh fruit as a treat, and drank only

THE GLYCEMIC INDEX

The glycemic index (GI) was initially developed in 1979 by scientists at the University of Toronto and Oxford University in England, to help diabetics make better food choices. Since then, scientists at the University of Sydney in Australia have carried out a significant amount of research on the subject and have established an international database of foods and their GI rankings at www.glycemicindex.com.

The index ranks foods according to how quickly a human body converts the carbohydrate in the food into glucose in the blood. Each food is tested on approximately 10 people, and their blood is tested several times during the next two hours to measure the effect of the carbohydrate in the food on their blood sugar. All this is done in a controlled lab setting to get an accurate measure of a food's speed of conversion to blood glucose. The more rapidly a food converts, the higher it raises levels of blood glucose.

Each food is assigned a numerical GI rating, from 0 to 100, based on its impact on blood sugar. Pure glucose, as a food, is given a value of 100 and is used as a reference point. The index is used only for foods that contain a significant amount of carbohydrates.

Although precise numeric GI rankings of individual foods are useful to scientists and perhaps dieticians in medical settings, they aren't practical tools for day-to-day life. Consequently, foods are generally grouped into low-, medium- and high-GI rankings. Low-GI foods do the best job at keeping blood-sugar levels stable, but that doesn't mean you can never eat foods with a higher GI ranking. Rather, by understanding a bit about how different foods impact your body, you can make wiser choices.

pure water or unsweetened herbal tea, the whole issue of GI ratings and blood-sugar control would become very simple. However, few people can live that way in our culture, and an approach to eating that is, in reality, impossible to sustain isn't very helpful.

Fortunately, it's quite possible to develop a style of eating that keeps blood-sugar levels stable, helps to balance hormones and promotes overall health and well-being. To accomplish those goals, you need to learn enough about food and beverages to discover which ones will both support your body well and give you a little pleasure as you eat them. Forcing yourself to eat and drink things you don't like will add stress to your life, which is counterproductive, and you won't be able to stick with your own program.

The glycemic index has been studied extensively around the world and several thousand studies and scientific articles have been published on the subject. Although there is still some debate in the medical community about its value, a significant body of research shows that, in addition to keeping hormones balanced, eating a low-GI diet reduces the chances of heart disease, diabetes and weight gain.

CHOOSING CARBOHYDRATES WISELY

It's possible to make a low-GI diet a complicated affair, but it isn't necessary. In talking about foods that raise blood sugar more or less quickly, we'll use the terms low GI, medium GI and high GI, since these terms are brief and widely used. The key thing is to get a sense of how various foods work, rather than focusing on exact categories or labels.

There is another important element. Many times, we eat a combination of foods rather than just one, such as cereal and milk, a sandwich, salad and chicken with garlic bread, or pasta with meat, seafood, sauce and/or vegetables. After any meal or snack, the degree to which blood sugar rises is influenced by the combination rather than a single food. Fat and protein slow down digestion, and when combined with high-GI carbohydrates, will also slow down their impact on blood sugar.

That said, you might be wondering, why bother looking at GI of individual carbohydrates? Why not just always eat carbohydrates with fat or protein, or both? You could do that if controlling blood sugar were the only goal of all the food you eat, but that becomes more restrictive and not completely practical. Like any artificial regimen, it isn't an approach that's likely to last. By gaining some familiarity with how different carbohydrates affect blood sugar, you're free to make your own choices and have an unlimited variety of foods at your disposal. If you don't find food very interesting, there is another benefit to becoming carbohydrate smart rather than restrictive: Eating a broader variety of nutritious foods will make your body healthier than restricting yourself to a few "safe" choices, even if all those choices are healthy ones.

The following list will give you an idea of which foods have low-, medium- or high-GI rankings, based on values obtained from the database at www.glycemicindex.com.

- Most vegetables are almost zero GI. Root vegetables, except potatoes, are usually low to medium GI.
- Fruits that grow in northern or Mediterranean climates are low-GI foods, whereas tropical fruits tend to rank a bit higher, mostly in the medium range.
- Bigger portions of higher-GI foods will raise blood sugar more than smaller ones.
- Traditional rolled oats (not instant oats), muesli (a granola-like wholegrain-nut-seed cereal originally from Switzerland) and bran cereals are low GI, whereas most regular U.S. breakfast cereals are high GI.
- White and whole wheat breads have the same high GI, in any form, including slices, buns, bagels, rolls, croissants and scones.
- Sourdough breads have a low GI because acidity slows the digestion of the grain.
- Dense breads made with whole grains other than wheat and those made with spelt flour have a low or medium GI.
- Potatoes, including french fries, are generally high GI. However, a potato salad made with vinegar and allowed to sit in the fridge will have a lower GI because the vinegar slows absorption.
- Acidic ingredients, such as balsamic vinegar used to dip bread, will generally reduce GI of carbohydrates.
- Pasta, white or whole wheat, has a low to medium GI, lower when cooked al dente (so that it's firm rather than soft). However, it should be eaten in small quantities, such as one serving described on food labels, which is much less than "normal" portions.

- Nuts and seeds are low GI.
- Both brown and white rice have a high GI. Basmati rice is medium GI. Quinoa and pearled barley make side dishes with a lower GI.
- Beans and legumes, such as lentils and peas, are very low GI. Baked beans usually contain sugar and are somewhat higher GI.
- Milk (any fat content) and plain yogurt are low GI. Flavored yogurt will be higher but should still be in the low to medium range.
- Fruit and vegetable juices have a somewhat higher GI than the foods they are extracted from because fiber, which has been removed from the juice, slows digestion. However, these beverages are still in the low to medium range.
- Any sweetened sodas or other sugary drinks, except for diet versions with no-calorie sweeteners, have a high GI, unless they also contain fat, such as high-calorie coffee or chocolate drinks. Tea, coffee and plain soda or mineral water have no effect on blood sugar. Plain water, soda and mineral water, with a spritz of citrus for flavor, will also have a near-zero effect on blood sugar.

If you prefer to check GI rankings without having to search an online database, *Transitions Lifestyle System Easy-to-Use Glycemic Index Food Guide* is a handy reference. A small paperback book that's easy to take with you to the supermarket, it can help you avoid foods and beverages that send your blood sugar on a roller-coaster ride.

4

FOOD TRAPS

Diets make seductive promises, and we want to believe them. Unfortunately, the chances of sticking with any diet for the longer term are slim to none, because the whole concept is built to fail. "Diet" has come to mean a regimented, artificially imposed set of restrictions for eating, excluding certain foods or severely limiting entire categories of food, such as carbohydrates in the case of low-carb diets.

The underlying premise is that the author of the diet knows what's best for our bodies and has invented or discovered a special way of manipulating food choices to bring about a different result than we normally get from eating. The whole thing can take on an almost magical quality, but it's not a sustainable way of life.

Eating to restore hormonal balance doesn't involve a diet in this present-day sense. Rather, it's more closely related to the origin of the word, which comes from the Greek diaita, meaning "manner of living." Instead of becoming subservient to a diet guru and giving up your power of choice over food, hormonal harmony starts with developing your own style of eating, based on an understanding of how various foods will influence your hormones and your overall state of health.

Managing carbohydrates is a basic principle, but other components also need to be taken into account: fats that help or hurt, ingredients that are hallmarks of havoc-wreaking foods, ingredients that are considered healthy but may not be right for you and often-overlooked foods that can promote overall good health and help to restore harmony. Controlling weight is also important because excess body fat contributes to hormonal imbalance by encouraging insulin resistance, and it promotes inflammation, increasing risk for heart disease, diabetes and cancer. With so many failures of weight-loss diets, the subject of weight control has become a very sensitive issue, but with a sensible approach that addresses the underlying mechanism of weight gain, it's possible to lose body fat and keep it off.

BLOOD SUGAR, APPETITE AND WEIGHT

In addition to disrupting hormonal balance, high-GI carbohydrates play a pivotal role in weight gain by tricking the body into mistakenly thinking it's starving. Several hours after a meal that causes blood-sugar levels to rapidly spike, the physiological response in a human body is the same as it would be after many hours of eating absolutely nothing. Not surprisingly, the body's response is "give me more food, right now," which manifests as irresistible hunger. Not only that, but there is most likely going to be a physical urge to eat more high-GI foods, especially among people who are already overweight. In short, this is a vicious cycle: Eat high-GI foods, get ravenously hungry within a few hours, crave more high-GI foods, on and on.

Many people try to lose weight by eating little or nothing all day long, but by dinner time, they are so uncontrollably hungry that they eat and eat and eat until bedtime. At that point, willpower or rational food choices go by the boards because insatiable hunger takes over as a survival mechanism, and to a body that feels threatened with starvation, high-calorie food is much more valuable than lower-calorie fare, regardless of its nutritional merit. And, it's impossible for anyone in this situation to think about portion control, which is a basic requirement for weight loss. This is another vicious cycle because the next morning, people in this situation usually have no appetite and again, eat little or nothing until uncontrollable hunger takes over towards the end of the day.

Falling prey to either one of these cycles doesn't mean you're genetically challenged, unintelligent, weak-willed or suffer from some other character flaw. It simply means that your body did not get the fuel it needed because you ate the wrong food or no food, and eventually, your body took matters into its own hands in an effort to survive.

There is a tried and tested way to break the vicious cycles: eating foods that slowly increase blood-sugar levels and keep them stable. Lab tests of people's responses to different types of meals throughout the day show that breakfast sets the stage for the entire day. If breakfast consists of foods that produce a slow and steady increase in blood sugar, the effects of later meals will not be as pronounced in terms of blood-sugar ups and downs and cravings.

As an example, if you eat low-GI eggs or rolled oats for breakfast, and drink water, or tea or coffee (preferably without caffeine), which are also low GI, your blood-sugar levels will rise gradually and remain stable for a few hours. If you eat a cookie before lunch (not recommended), your blood sugar will spike, but less so than if you had eaten a doughnut or sugary cereal with soda for breakfast. In other words, eating sugary, starchy food first thing in the morning sets you up for a pattern of ups and downs in energy levels, cravings for more unhealthy foods, an appetite that is out of control, weight gain and disruption of hormone balance. Breakfast really is the most important meal of the day.

NUTRITIOUS VS. EMPTY CALORIES

Nutritious foods contain, per calorie, a significant amount of beneficial nutrients that promote good health, hormonal balance and well-being. In contrast, foods with empty calories contain few nutrients, leaving you wanting more, promoting weight gain and poor health. The foods you eat should nourish your body and make you feel good, and only those with nutritious calories, such as vegetables, fruits, nuts, whole grains, beans and legumes, fish, poultry and meats that are lean and unprocessed, can do the job. Calorie-rich foods, such as refined breads, pastries and cookies, french fries, fatty meats and sauces, lead to weight gain while disrupting hormones, reducing energy levels, damaging arteries and causing digestive problems.

Timing food is also critical. Eating small amounts of low-GI foods every three hours or so is more effective in keeping blood-sugar levels stable than eating larger meals less frequently. When your body doesn't go into starvation mode and hunger is controllable, it's quite realistic to make conscious choices of healthy foods while keeping portions small. If you've never tried this approach, it may seem counterintuitive but it works like a charm. Small, frequent meals or snacks of low-GI foods provide a steady stream of energy, reduce stress and result in fuel (calories from food) going to muscles rather than fat, thereby contributing to a leaner body. In terms of food, if a magic bullet exists, this is it.

HARMFUL AND HELPFUL FATS

Fats can work for you or against you, depending on their quantity and quality. Fat is digested gradually and slows down the digestion of other food with which it is consumed. When you eat carbohydrates with fat, the conversion of carbohydrates to blood sugar occurs at a slower rate. This can be beneficial by tempering spikes in blood sugar. However, if you eat too much fat in any given meal, the fat content can interfere with the function of insulin, making it more difficult for the insulin to deliver the carbohydrate calories to muscle cells. Using the pizza analogy in chapter 2, you could think of an overabundance of fat acting like bad weather, engine trouble or very deep potholes when a pizza delivery guy is driving to a home in the muscle cell neighborhood. Eating some, but not too much fat at any given meal is what works best.

Choosing high-quality fat is just as important as moderating quantity. Healthy fats, such as those from fish, olive oil and flax-seed, are necessary for the function of every cell. They reduce inflammation; help to balance hormones and reduce risk for heart disease, diabetes, and inflammatory diseases such as arthritis; support healthy function of the brain and nervous system; and protect against mood swings and depression. Fish oil, in supplements or in fish, is particularly beneficial as it improves insulin function, blunts inflammation, helps to control weight and may relieve menstrual pain. Saturated fats in meats and dairy products need to be eaten in moderation. However, there is one type of fat, trans fat, that is deadly, and the human body has absolutely no physiological need for it.

TRANS FAT

Nutrition and medical experts almost never recommend virtually eliminating any type of food from our diets, but trans fat is an exception. The only manmade fat that is prevalent in our diets, trans fat is produced through a chemical process, using hydrogen, which converts liquid oils to solids. The processing extends shelf life and produces a fat that is easy to use for deep frying. In processed foods, such as packaged pastries and cookies, trans fat creates a certain texture that people have come to expect. On ingredient labels, trans fats are usually listed as "partially hydrogenated" oils or "shortening."

To be technically accurate, there is a type of trans fat that occurs naturally in red meat and dairy products, but its chemical structure is different from manmade trans fat. The natural form occurs in miniscule quantities, and studies have not found it to be harmful.

In fact, some research suggests that the natural form may offer some benefit. In a nutshell, no one in the scientific or medical communities is concerned about naturally occurring trans fats.

All the news coverage about trans fats, as the term is used day to day, refers to the manmade form, which is a health hazard. A significant body of research shows that these types of fats raise the risk for heart disease because they increase "bad" LDL cholesterol, lower "good" HDL cholesterol, and make arteries less flexible and more constricted. And, they increase risk for diabetes. A study published in the *New England Journal of Medicine* estimated that up to 19 percent of heart disease in the United States, or 228,000 cases per year, might be averted if trans fats were reduced to near-zero levels in our food supply.

Why does anyone add trans fats to food? For the most part, it's become a matter of convenience for food manufacturers. America has been eating this dangerous type of fat since 1911 when Crisco shortening, the first trans fat product, appeared on store shelves. During World War II, butter was in short supply, and margarine, made of trans fat, became a popular substitute. Then, in the 1950s, we learned that saturated fat was unhealthy, so trans fats replaced various forms of saturated fat in baked and packaged foods, and partially hydrogenated oils became the standard for restaurant deep frying.

It wasn't until the 1990s that researchers began discovering the risks of trans fats, and as evidence grew, health advocates started lobbying for these fats to be eliminated from restaurant deep fryers. In the late 1990s, the U.S. government began proposing legislation to list trans fat content of food labels, but no new laws were passed for some years.

THE TRANS FAT LABEL TRAP

Since 2006, trans fat content has been listed on nutrition labels of packaged foods, but labels can be misleading. By law, if a food contains 0.5 grams (which is the same as 500 mg) or more trans fat per serving, the trans fat quantity must be stated on the Nutrition Facts panel, the same part of the label that lists calories, fat, protein, etc. If one serving of a food contains anything less than 0.5 grams, such as 0.4 grams or even 0.49 grams, by law, the quantity of trans fat is stated as 0 g (grams). If the ingredients list includes partially hydrogenated oils or shortening, it indicates that some trans fats are present in the food.

Less than half a gram doesn't sound like much, but it is. If you eat several servings of a food, or several foods with 0.4 grams of trans fat in each (listed as 0 g of trans fats on the labels), it's easy to accumulate several grams of trans fats in a day, and in the case of these types of fats, that's a significant quantity.

An analysis of several studies that examined the impact of trans fats on nearly 140,000 people found this: increasing daily intake of trans fats by a mere 2 percent increased heart disease by 23 percent. Other research found that people who ate the most trans fats tripled their risk of sudden death from heart disease. If you find it difficult to connect with numbers, it might help to understand what our bodies do with trans fats.

Keep in mind that we're talking about a fat that has never existed in nature, so it's a foreign substance which cannot be utilized like other food by the cells that make up our bodies. Each cell has a membrane that houses receptors, including insulin receptors (doors to the houses in the pizza delivery analogy). Trans fats disrupt the health of these membranes, thereby upsetting the function of each cell. If you imagine a door that is coming off its hinges and no longer fits or opens and closes properly, that's sort of what happens to cell membranes as a result of trans fats.

Based on scientific evidence, the American Heart Association (AHA) recommends some specific daily limits for trans fats, stated as no more than 1 percent of calories. This is what it means in practical terms: If you eat approximately 2,000 calories per day, an amount that few people need to exceed, the trans fat limit recommended by the AHA would be about 2 grams. It's calculated this way: One percent of 2,000 calories is 20 calories. Fat contains 9 calories per gram, and 20 divided by 9 is 2.2. If you eat about 1,500 calories daily, the trans fat limit would be approximately 1.6 grams, and for 1,200 calories daily, trans fats shouldn't exceed approximately 1.3 grams.

How much trans fat might you be eating on a regular basis? Unless you know for a fact that a restaurant (a fast-food outlet or any other type of restaurant) does not use trans fat, one fried chicken dinner, a large order of fries or a baked dessert could contain anywhere from 7 to 15 grams of trans fats. Cookies, buns, sweet or savory pies (such as chicken pot pies), and other baked or processed foods with partially hydrogenated oil or shortening in the ingredient list—even if the Nutrition Facts panel says 0 grams of trans fats—could give you just short of half a gram per serving. Given that servings are frequently smaller than amounts typically eaten, you could easily be eating one or more grams of trans fats in any food with "Trans Fats 0 g." If a food lists a specified quantity of trans fats, do the math.

Practically speaking, it's probably easier to avoid trans fats than trying to keep your intake below 2 grams or so. You can stay trans fat-free in restaurants by skipping fried and baked goods, likely sources of trans fats, and instead, ordering grilled meat, poultry or fish (without batter) and raw, steamed or grilled vegetables. In supermarkets, you can find convenient foods without partially hydrogenated oils or shortening. Try reading ingredient labels of foods in your cupboards and refrigerator, then, next time you shop, look for alternatives without trans fats.

You might be wondering why trans fats aren't banned completely. The City of New York did ban them from being used in restaurants, and other cities have followed since then. But beyond that, the answer is somewhat complex. Because trans fats are so pervasive in our food supply, removing them requires changing the processes for manufacturing thousands of foods. Efforts to replace trans fats with healthier ingredients have been ongoing during the past few years, but in the meantime, it's up to you to make wise choices. By buying healthier foods, you're letting restaurants, stores and food manufacturers know which path they should be taking while improving your own well-being.

HALLMARKS OF FOOD QUALITY

Higher quality, nutritious food is less likely to contain trans fats and another popular ingredient: high fructose corn syrup. While experts agree that trans fats are undesirable, high fructose corn syrup is much more controversial. Some science seems to support the idea that the sweetener is metabolized in a way that poses health risks and has contributed to an epidemic of obesity and diabetes, while other research draws opposite conclusions. Scientific controversy aside, there are economic reasons why the sweetener is found is almost any type of processed food, including sodas, ketchup, sauces, soups, breads, cookies, pastries and virtually any type of canned, frozen or other packaged food.

High fructose corn syrup began to be used widely in the 1980s. Manufactured from corn using a chemical process (it's not the same thing as plain old corn syrup), it was cheaper than sugar, making it profitable for soda manufacturers to offer super-sized drinks for lower prices. By helping to popularize oversized sodas, the sweetener has definitely contributed to expanding waistlines, insulin resistance and hormone disruption.

In addition to adding sweetness, high fructose corn syrup improves the shelf life and texture of food. Consequently, it's found in many foods that aren't desserts, because it makes it easier for food manufacturers to produce convenient foods that appeal to your taste buds. However, the rest of your body, including your hormones, may not respond so well to these foods because they are generally nutrient poor and rich in empty calories. As with trans fats, eliminating high fructose corn syrup from your diet will put you on a healthier track and help to restore hormonal balance.

On the positive side, these are some of the key foods and ingredients that contribute to your health: rolled oats; eggs (free range or omega-3 enriched are best); any amount of non-starchy vegetables; small amounts of yams or sweet potatoes rather than white potatoes; high-fiber fruits such as apples, pears and berries; olive oil; fish; flaxseed oil; vinegars; low-sodium marinades; whole grains such as quinoa; breads made with whole grains other than wheat; herbal teas; filtered water; garlic; a variety of spices; honey; lean meat; and skinless poultry.

When you're eating out, look for restaurants that serve meat, poultry and fish that is grilled or baked without batter or breading; grilled or steamed vegetables; salads that are really fresh, delicious and served with vinaigrette dressings rather than creamy ones; and offer a menu that uses some imagination instead of relying on fat to make tasty dishes. The same elements work for take-out. Consumer demand is driving the growth of healthier foods, and they're becoming more widely available in both stores and restaurants.

Working out a healthy, hormone-balancing way of eating that suits your own tastes and lifestyle requires more effort at first, but then it becomes second nature. Initially, simply reading a lot of food labels can take some time, but once you've found healthy versions of things you like to eat and drink, you'll settle into a new routine, one that makes you feel much better.

5

RESTORING HARMONY WITH FOOD

Before you put something in your mouth,
think about what it's doing for your energy,
your vitality and your good looks.

—JACK LALANNE, AT AGE 93

Back in the days when people relied on hunting and gathering skills to put food in their mouths, selecting nutritious food was simple. Everything was natural and fresh, and packages didn't exist. No one needed to read complicated food labels or worry about how much refined flour, sugar or fat they were eating, although they did have to watch out for wild beasts and poisonous plants. Granted, "shopping" for a meal wasn't exactly convenient, but then again, exercise "on the go" made up for the lack of health clubs.

Fast forward to a supermarket today: It may be convenient, but choosing foods that make a body feel good is far from simple because the beasts are disguised and neatly packaged. However, packages do provide a bit of guidance in a very simple sense, much more so than details on labels. Essentially, fresh foods should constitute the majority of the edible stuff that goes into your shopping cart, whereas packaged food should make up the minority.

Stop and think about that for a moment. It isn't the way most people shop. It may not seem convenient. It may seem ludicrous, even laughable. But guess what, it's a very basic way to sift through the mind-boggling options in any supermarket. Laugh, sigh or spit at the page if you must, but be willing to contemplate how this way of eating might work, at least to some extent.

Maybe the idea of eating mostly fresh food makes perfect sense but doesn't seem practical. So, let's see how we can make it work. It's helpful to prioritize which foods are most important in helping you achieve and maintain hormonal harmony, stay free of common chronic diseases and, best of all, maintain a physical state that enables you to enjoy life and live it the way you think you should. People often change the way they eat when confronted with a serious medical diagnosis, but there's no reason to wait until something life-threatening rears its head. If your hormones are going wild, that's a good reason to make changes. But even if you're only experiencing subtle symptoms or you just want to avoid discomfort down the road, the prospect of a better way to live is always good motivation.

TOP PRIORITIES

There are several things that food should do to restore and maintain harmony among hormones:

- Keep blood-sugar levels stable.
- Decrease inflammation.
- Provide sustained energy.
- Help you to reduce body fat if you're overweight.

- Help you to maintain a healthy weight.
- Contribute to your overall health and well-being.
- Reduce risk for chronic diseases such as diabetes, heart disease, cancer and osteoporosis.
- Keep your taste buds happy.

The last one is just as important as the others, if not more so, because if a healthy food doesn't taste good to you, it will get replaced by an unhealthy one.

TAKING CARE OF TASTE BUDS

If you are accustomed to eating processed or fast food on a regular basis, your taste buds may not be thrilled with healthier food at first. Both processed and fast foods are usually high in salt and fat, rather than being seasoned with a greater variety of spices, and may use strong artificial flavors to disguise lack of flavor in the underlying food. Nature didn't design fresh food to last for months or years on store shelves, and when convenience becomes a priority, food manufacturers have to make some alterations. Healthy, freshly prepared food tastes different.

In a sense, processed foods overwhelm and desensitize taste buds. Just as ear drums become desensitized after being close to a speaker at a rock concert, taste buds tend to become somewhat deadened by large amounts of salt, fat and artificial flavors, and may not immediately detect or appreciate nature's flavors. It's important to allow your mouth to discover a whole new panorama of tastes.

Assuming you don't overcook things, quality and freshness of food will exert the biggest influence on how much it appeals to your mouth. To please your taste buds in a healthy way, these are some things to keep in mind when buying and preparing food.

BUY THE FRESHEST PRODUCE you can find. When produce has to travel long distances after being harvested, it has to be picked before becoming ripe, which means the natural flavor hasn't had time to fully develop. Locally grown vegetables and fruits can be picked at their prime and should have more flavor. Find stores in your area that buy from local farms and shop at farmers markets whenever possible. In stores, feel free to ask for samples before buying fresh produce.

NEVER BUY FISH THAT SMELLS FISHY because the odor means it isn't fresh. Whenever you're not buying frozen fish or seafood, ask if there is any fresh (never frozen) fish that was delivered that day. Availability will vary, depending on where you live, but it pays to find out what is offered in your neighborhood. Ordering online is another option, although a more costly one.

BUY THE HIGHEST-QUALITY LEAN MEAT YOU CAN AFFORD.

INSTEAD OF ORDINARY TABLE SALT, use kosher; it brings out more flavor in food and contains less sodium.

TRY FRESH GROUND PEPPER and different herbs and spices to season grilled meats, fish and vegetables, including flavored sea salts which can have natural smoke or many other flavors with less sodium than ordinary table salt. For maximum taste and aroma, season with flavored salts and fresh pepper after food has been prepared.

FOR LEAN MEATS AND FISH, try marinating before grilling or baking. When buying marinades, choose ones that are low in sodium and free of artificial flavors and preservatives.

USE NON-STICK PANS AND GRILLS to cook with less added fat.

DON'T OVERCOOK VEGETABLES. To bring out natural flavors, steam vegetables lightly so that they are still somewhat crisp. Inexpensive steamer inserts that fit most pots are available in supermarkets and kitchen stores, or you can use steamer bags in a microwave, although the microwave gives you less control over the cooking process. And don't be afraid to grill vegetables.

TOP FOODS

We think of multitasking as a recent invention, but when it comes to food, nature has always worked this way. The best foods for controlling blood sugar and restoring hormonal balance also help to keep human beings lean; reduce inflammation and protect against heart disease, diabetes, cancer and osteoporosis; and help to bolster our immune system so that we are more resistant to bugs and viruses in our environment.

These are the top foods to incorporate into your diet.

FISH

Omega-3 fats found in coldwater fish are necessary for the healthy function of all cells. These fats are building blocks of cell membranes, the outer layers of cells which house receptors that accept fuel—in the form of glucose in the blood. By improving the health of cell membranes, omega-3 fats increase the ability of muscle cells to accept and use fuel to generate energy, improving blood-sugar levels and the efficiency of metabolism. By eating fish, you get these therapeutic fats along with healthy protein.

If you recall from the previous chapters, hormonal imbalance is triggered after we eat too many starchy, sugary refined foods, an overabundance of blood glucose is delivered to muscle cells and these cells become overwhelmed and eventually stop accepting the fuel. Insulin is the hormone that transports the blood glucose, and when the muscle cells resist its attempts to deliver the fuel, the condition is called insulin resistance. Omega-3 fats are a key tool for reversing and preventing insulin resistance, and by doing so, they help to restore hormonal balance. They also support healthy weight loss.

Coldwater fish is the richest source of omega-3 fats. Other benefits of eating this type of fish include significantly lower risk for heart disease, stroke and diabetes, as well as improvements in skin, mood, arthritis and other inflammatory conditions and menstrual pain.

Salmon is the top source of omega-3 fats. As a rule, wild salmon contains larger amounts of the healthy fats than farmed varieties. Sardines and tuna are other rich sources, but albacore, the most popular type of tuna, is higher in mercury than the other options. Albacore is a very large fish with a longer lifespan than salmon or sardines, so it accumulates more mercury in its flesh. Canned "light" tuna usually comes from smaller varieties and contains less mercury. However, the benefits of eating albacore tuna occasionally may outweigh the liabilities of its mercury content. For sandwiches and salads, canned salmon is convenient and extremely beneficial.

Aim to eat coldwater fish two or three times a week.

FLAX

The oil in flaxseed is the richest plant source of omega-3 fats, and the seeds are a good source of fiber. Eating 1 to 2 tablespoons of flaxseed daily may help to reduce risk for heart disease and cancer. The omega-3 fats in flax occur in a different form than those in fish, and some argue that the flax version may not be utilized as well, but these fats in flaxseed are tremendously beneficial. If, on principle, you consume no animal foods, flax is a good source of omega-3 fats. And even if you eat fish, flax is a beneficial food to include in your routine diet.

Many people find that toasted flaxseeds add a pleasant crunch to salads, soups and sandwiches, and ground seeds can add body to smoothies. Flaxseed oil contains the highest concentration of the plant's omega-3 fats. It has a low smoke point and should not be used in cooking but can provide healthy fats in smoothies, salads and other foods.

NUTS

All types of nuts contain healthy fats and fiber that help to keep blood sugar stable. They also contain magnesium and potassium, which help to control blood pressure, and a host of other beneficial nutrients. Nuts help to reduce risk for heart disease and, when eaten as part of a healthy diet, can help to control appetite and weight.

When buying nuts, keep in mind that roasted nuts may also contain trans fats in oils used during the roasting process, which counters the benefits of eating the nuts. Check labels of roasted nuts and avoid partially hydrogenated oils. Raw nuts contain the most nutrients, and dry-roasted ones are the next best. A small handful of nuts or two tablespoons of a nut butter is all you need to reap some benefits while eating a reasonable amount of calories.

If you don't like raw nuts, sprinkle them with cinnamon, which also helps to regulate blood sugar, and roast them in your own oven. Your kitchen will smell good, and your nuts will be trans-fat-free and delicious. If you eat chips or other refined snack foods, it's a good idea to replace them with a small handful of nuts. Or, combine a few nuts or nut butter with an apple for a snack. Who said nut butter can only be eaten on crackers or bread?

LEAN PROTEIN

Virtually any type of lean protein will have a beneficial effect on blood sugar and help to reverse or prevent the insulin resistance that triggers hormonal imbalance. When it comes to any type of meat, lean cuts have fewer calories, are more nutrient dense and contain fewer toxins. Unless you eat organic meat, which is highly recommended, any hormones and antibiotics used in raising the animals, as well as pesticides in animal feed, will accumulate in the fat. Eggs are also a form of lean protein, and some are enriched with omega-3 fats. They're a nutritious and versatile food, and there's no reason not to eat them frequently.

Beef is one of our staples, but its nutritional profile varies quite a bit. By nature, cows eat grass, but corn has become the usual feed for American cows. Corn-fed beef is generally more tender, but it also contains more saturated fat and calories than grass-fed varieties, which have been gaining popularity in recent years. Grass-fed beef is better for you, because it is lower in saturated fat and may be a significant source of omega-3 fats, depending on the quality of its feed. Grass-fed beef costs more, and many people don't like its taste and texture, but it's certainly worth trying. If your local stores don't carry it, plenty of farmers sell direct online.

Lean beef and pork and skinless poultry are all good sources of protein. Game meats are leaner than corn-fed beef, but all too often, they're prepared with a lot of added, unhealthy fat. If you like game, marinating it overnight in spices and a little olive oil is a better option. Processed meats that are smoked, cured or prepared with salt or other preservatives, including bologna and other luncheon meats, increase risk for colorectal cancer.

Soy foods can be a meat alternative. If you eat anything other than traditional Asian soy foods, such as edamame, tofu or tempe, check ingredient labels to make sure there are no unhealthy ingredients, such as overly generous amounts of fat or preservatives, added to non-traditional, Western versions of soy products such as veggie burgers.

To minimize triggers of hormonal imbalance, include lean protein in every meal.

VEGETABLES

When it comes to vegetables, variety rules. Vegetables contain such a bounty of nutrients, scientists have barely begun to identify and understand them. But we do know this: among people who eat the same quantities of vegetables, those who eat a greater variety experience better health. Color is a good way to track the quality of your own diet because different colors come from different types of nutrients, so feel free to go wild in painting your own plate.

With the exceptions of potatoes, yams, sweet potatoes and starchy squashes, which should be eaten in moderation, the "all you can eat" principle works well for vegetables. Non-starchy vegetables contain fiber and a significant amount of water, both of which are filling, so it would be difficult to ingest enough calories from them to cause weight gain, and they don't cause spikes in blood sugar, so they don't induce food cravings. However, any vegetable can be turned into a high-fat, high-calorie food if it is fried or smothered in rich sauces or butter; avoid those pitfalls.

Based on a review of 7,000 studies, the American Institute for Cancer Research recommends that adults eat at least 14 ounces of non-starchy vegetables and fruits daily to reduce risk for cancer. Vegetables, along with fruits, are also beneficial for bones. Western diets tend to make the human body acidic, which increases excretion of calcium and weakens bones; vegetables and fruits are alkaline and reduce acidity, helping to preserve bones.

Fresh vegetables are best, but frozen ones run a close second. To avoid toxins, buy organic whenever possible. Eat vegetables raw in salads, lightly steamed or grilled.

FRUIT

Although fruit is another bountiful gift from nature, it can become too much of a good thing. Fruit contains natural sugars, which, when eaten to excess, can contribute to elevated blood sugar that leads to disrupted hormones. Apples and berries are the best choices for hormonal balance because they are high in fiber and have less impact on blood sugar than tropical fruits.

In studies, apples, in comparison to other fruit, have been most consistently linked with reduced risk for heart disease, cancer, asthma and type 2 diabetes, and they've also been found to improve memory and lung function and help to reduce weight. The peel contains two to six times the antioxidants of the flesh, depending on the variety. However, the peel is also where you'll find pesticide residues, and apples are one of the chief sources of pesticides in our diets. Buy organic, don't peel and enjoy.

Berries offer a higher concentration of antioxidants than most other foods, are associated with lower rates of cancer and heart disease and can quell inflammation. And they're delicious. When you can't get fresh ones, buy frozen and thaw them slowly in the microwave. When thawing, spread them out on a plate lined with paper towel, and they will seem almost like fresh berries.

LEGUMES AND WHOLE GRAINS

Legumes (beans, lentils and peas) and whole grains round out any meal. Both contain fiber, which slows down digestion and helps to keep blood-sugar levels stable, and a host of beneficial vitamins and minerals. People who regularly eat legumes and whole grains, in moderation, experience less heart disease, diabetes and cancer. As with vegetables, variety produces the greatest benefits, so experiment and find your own favorites.

EXTRA VIRGIN OLIVE OIL

While it isn't a source of omega-3 fats, olive oil contains other healthy fats that help to stabilize blood-sugar levels. Extra virgin olive oil (not lower grades of olive oil) contains significant levels of antioxidants and helps to lower blood pressure, increase "good" HDL cholesterol, reduce inflammation, prevent cancer and may fight H. pylori bacteria that cause stomach ulcers. Extra virgin olive oil is obtained from the first pressing of olives and is the highest quality. The lower grades, called "virgin olive oil," "pure olive oil" or simply "olive oil," are typically used in frying as they have a higher smoke point.

Extra virgin olive oil is delicious for dipping and is better for you than butter. It makes a great dressing for salads and adds flavor when drizzled on raw or cooked vegetables.

VINEGARS

The acidity in vinegar reduces the speed at which carbohydrates are absorbed, which helps to curb spikes in blood-sugar levels, reduce cravings and keep hormones in sync. The tremendous variety of vinegars available today means a lot of flavor choices. Take advantage of any opportunity to sample different ones at food fairs or in gourmet stores. Vinegars can be used in marinades, sauces and dips as well as in salad dressings.

PITFALLS TO AVOID

LIQUID SUGAR

Sodas and other sugary drinks, such as fruit, sports or energy drinks, can wreak havoc with your weight, blood sugar and hormones. There's only one way to deal with the problem: Drink something else. Good choices are filtered water (without artificial flavoring) and caffeine-free herbal teas.

If you like flavored water, add a spritz of fresh lemon, orange or lime, or add cucumber slices. If you dislike herbal teas without sweeteners, try adding a little agave syrup, which is a flavorful and slowly absorbed natural sweetener. To wean yourself off sugary beverages, replace them gradually with healthier options, one glass, can or bottle at a time.

ZERO-CALORIE SWEETENERS

Contrary to popular belief, zero-calorie sweeteners in diet drinks can promote weight gain. In an article in the *Journal of the American Medical Association*, one researcher summed up study results this way: "Although low-calorie sweeteners are a dietary staple for many individuals trying to maintain or lose weight, an emerging body of evidence suggests these substances offer little help to dieters and may even help promote weight gain." It appears that artificial zero-calorie sweeteners may trick the brain into expecting more calories, thereby promoting desire for sweet foods. Aspartame, a popular but controversial sweetener, has been linked with abdominal cramps, headaches, dizziness and many other symptoms.

No one really knows the exact implications of these sweeteners on hormone balance, but given the evidence so far, it makes sense to avoid them.

DAIRY FOODS

Milk, cheese, yogurt and other dairy foods are slowly absorbed sources of various nutrients, including calcium and vitamin D, but many people don't tolerate dairy foods well and experience digestive problems that may not seem related. If your digestion is not what you'd like it to be, try reducing or eliminating dairy foods and see if you feel better.

WHEAT AND GLUTEN

Wheat, whether whole or refined, is a rapidly absorbed carbohydrate, whereas other grains are absorbed more slowly and are better options for hormonal balance. In addition, many people have difficulty digesting wheat, and some cannot digest gluten, a component of most grains. If you have digestive problems, try eliminating wheat–or all grains–for a while to see if it could be the culprit.

FOOD SENSITIVITIES

For some people, perfectly healthy foods can cause an adverse reaction that isn't an obvious food allergy. Generally referred to as a food sensitivity, these types of reactions are usually delayed. Someone might feel tired or inexplicably gain weight and the food connection may be hard to identify, but when that food is eliminated, good health returns. Testing for these types of food reactions is typically available through physicians who take an integrative approach to healing.

EVERY BIT COUNTS

It's easy to underestimate the impact of seemingly minor

changes in how we live. For example, you might think it takes quite a bit of extra food to gain 10 pounds but consider this: Eating 100 calories more than you burn, every single day, will produce a gain of slightly more than 10 pounds in one year, nearly 21 pounds in two years, and so on. The change could be something as simple as eating an extra cookie or two each day. Or, on the activity side of the equation, it could result from moving from an office where you frequently walked up and down stairs during the work day to one where there are no stairs.

It's unlikely that anyone habitually eats exactly 100 extra calories daily. However, it is realistic to start making significant health improvements with small changes, one at a time. Just as small bricks can be used to build a big wall, small changes can eventually add up to a whole new lease on life.

6

STRESS LESS

I'm late, I'm late, for a very important date.

—THE WHITE RABBIT

Why is that line from *Alice in Wonderland* so memorable? Well, it was uttered by a rabbit and talking animals are cute, but also, the scene captures a feeling we're all too familiar with: being under stress. It's a universal human experience, and without it we couldn't survive.

The human body's stress response is designed to be an asset. It enables us to muster our resources, physically and mentally, to overcome danger or other, unexpected challenges. Our entire system goes on alert and, temporarily, functions at peak capacity. If you've ever scaled an inhospitable mountain or gone the proverbial extra mile to accomplish some seemingly impossible task, your body's stress response helped you succeed. However, that same stress response becomes a liability when it's activated for long periods of time or becomes chronically jammed in high gear.

In times of stress, the body produces extra cortisol. If this happens for a short period followed by recovery, a healthy person will be able to take it in stride, but if it becomes an ongoing situation, the extra cortisol production throws other hormones out of balance. In addition, the adrenal glands, which produce cortisol, can become overworked, eventually leading to adrenal fatigue. At that point, the adrenal glands are unable to produce adequate cortisol, resulting in persistent low levels of energy, especially in the morning, and possibly other symptoms, including unexplained weight gain or loss, respiratory problems and a predisposition to other illnesses.

When the adrenal glands don't function properly, thyroid function is also impaired. The thyroid gland produces thyroid hormones that—in simple terms—drive metabolism. However, to work properly, the thyroid needs assistance from the adrenal glands. As an analogy, if the adrenal glands are weak, the thyroid hormone is like an engine revving with the transmission in park. When such situations continue, thyroid hormone levels can eventually become depleted, and if the thyroid is treated before adrenal function is repaired, a person will feel worse.

Controlling cortisol, by managing the triggers of stress, is a key to hormonal balance and overall health. Eating too many sugary, starchy carbohydrates is one trigger of cortisol overproduction. Other triggers include stressful life situations, too much or too little exercise, and toxins, which are covered in the next chapter. Managing these factors in a sensible way can work wonders by decreasing stress, maintaining healthy levels of cortisol and restoring well-being and hormonal balance.

PEOPLE

Occasional stress is part and parcel of human interaction, but we generally have the ability to make some choices that influence our own stress levels. We can't control everything that comes our way but most often, we have more than one option in terms of reacting to a given situation.

Our most stressful relationships, whether at home or at work, usually revolve around one, or a very few people. In each case, it takes two to tangle. You probably know what irritates the other individual and what he or she does that irritates you. The next time you have an opportunity to do something irritating, try not doing it and see what happens.

Think of it this way: A wet towel helps to douse flames, whereas gasoline makes them rage. Ceasing to say or do things that we know irritate the other person acts much like a wet towel and can defuse many potentially explosive situations. This does not mean you should let people walk all over you, but you can probably be a bit more responsible for your own actions. If you reach a point where you just want to scream at someone, step away for a moment, determine what it is that you really want to communicate and figure out a way to get your point across in a calm, rational and simple manner

Some situations, especially those you can't escape, may also require another strategy: setting boundaries. As an example, let's say your source of stress is your mother. Start by evaluating how she creates stress and work out a way to limit her ability to do so in those particular arenas. If she calls almost daily and talks endlessly about her 20-year-old feud with Aunt Tillie, try something along these lines: Calmly tell her you love her but you need to limit your phone calls with her to 30 minutes twice a week and if she begins to rehash her upset with Aunt Tillie, you'll have to stop the conversation. And keep your promise.

The same strategies can smooth out work stress. For example, if you are overworked because your boss is continually putting an unrealistic number of projects on your plate, try this type of approach: Determine how many projects you can realistically handle at one time and tell your boss. Write the name of each project on an index card, pin the cards on a corkboard system on the wall and clearly mark any available spaces for additional projects on the board. When your boss comes along with another project, write it down on a new index card and ask him or her to remove the card with the "extra" project you need to stop working on to make room for the new one. It's quite possible that your boss had no idea how much you accomplish and this way, you both have a clear picture of what you are working on at any given time.

Stress is reduced when you feel you have some control and are being heard. In both of the examples above, taking a wet towel approach while setting boundaries enables you to reclaim some of your power and be an advocate for yourself without creating drama or feeding the fire. The most important thing is to give yourself enough respect to rationally set your boundaries and maintain your energy and strength.

Some personal or business relationships are simply toxic, and the only way you can escape the stress they cause is by distancing yourself. If this isn't realistic, at least in the short term, the strategies above will help. In addition, you can minimize stress in other areas of your life. One way is to exercise any power of choice you do have regarding the rest of the people you allow into your life.

Joy is contagious. That fact is not only intuitive but also scientifically proven. In a study of more than 4,000 people, researchers found that happiness spreads in a chain reaction among people who are socially connected. They calculated that you're 15 percent more likely to be happy if directly connected to a happy person; 10 percent if it's the friend of a friend who is happy; and 6 percent if it's the friend of a friend of a friend who is happy. Unhappiness also spreads, but to a lesser extent.

TIME

Time can seem like a scarce commodity because it's easy to lose track of how it's being spent, even with the best of intentions. Consider this: An hour of TV per day adds up to 15 days and nights plus 5 hours in one year. If you consider a day as the 16 hours when you're not sleeping, the daily TV hour adds up to nearly 23 days. Increasing TV time to 1.5 hours per day brings the total to more than a month, or more precisely, 34 days plus 3.5 hours. This is simply an example, not an attempt to condemn home entertainment. The math is the same for any hour-long daily activity, such as commuting to work or driving kids around.

Lack of time is considered "normal" in our culture. If you pay attention to popular media, it would seem that having an over-booked schedule is a desirable, politically correct way to live, because it means you have an active, vibrant life. There's a glitch in such logic. Being productive and being stressed are two different things, and in fact, being chronically under stress will make you less productive while disrupting your hormones and predisposing you to disease.

Prioritizing what you do, day to day, is a key to reducing time stress. On one hand, there may be extraneous tasks you do that aren't really necessary, and on the other, there may be things you should be doing for your own well-being that need to be added to your schedule.

Women are particularly prone to putting other people's needs ahead of their own, thinking that it's selfish to put themselves first. If that describes you, keep in mind that by enhancing your own state of wellness, you will be able to make a more valuable contribution to the lives of others. If it seems counterintuitive, think of a day when you felt exceptionally good and look back at how that affected the people in your life. Imagine how things could be if you were at your best all or most of the time.

Unless you feel that your stress level is very low, it's a good idea to take a look at your daily routine. See if there are extraneous tasks you are neither obligated nor personally compelled to take on, and make some changes. Getting enough sleep, preferably at least eight hours each night, is a basic necessity.

In addition, realize that you need some time to yourself and add some "me time" to your schedule. What will you do with that time? It should be something you like, something that helps you unwind and leaves you feeling rejuvenated, or at least relaxed. If simply thinking about finding "me time" makes you feel stressed, don't panic. Aim for five minutes to start and build from there. Pretend you have to brush your teeth one extra time during the day but use those minutes for something you enjoy.

Some people find that specific meditation practices are effective anti-stress tools, but different things work for each of us. The objective is to do something that soothes you, to step aside from the day and take a breather. It could be going for a walk, reading your favorite magazine or a good book, doing a little gardening, taking a leisurely bath, window shopping, rearranging furniture or pictures on the wall, sketching, calling an old friend, sitting down in your favorite chair and looking out the window or sitting on a rock in your garden and counting blades of grass. This is about doing something that boosts your spirits. If you work outside your home, try changing your routine during your lunch hour or take a break, if only for five or ten minutes, and go for a walk.

Remember, the stress response is a good thing only when it helps us to survive during a temporary moment of danger or crisis and, most importantly, is followed by a recovery that allows us to get back to normal. One or more little breaks in your day can help to keep you out of a damaging state of chronic stress and help to restore and maintain hormonal balance.

MONEY

Money can be a source of stress that often boils down to differing opinions about how to spend or save it, who was responsible for causing a financial difficulty, how to make more or, in the case of a divorce, how much goes to each party. All these situations can contribute to hormonal disruption, which in turn clouds judgment and makes it even more difficult to work out a solution.

Keep in mind that money is a tool. If you can use it wisely to help keep yourself in a state of wellness, it will be easier to resolve financial difficulties.

When money seems scarce, either because your personal finances truly are strained or because economic news is gloomy, it's easy to turn to comfort foods that, in reality, provide anything but comfort. Because they are generally starchy, sugary and high in fat, comfort foods are the perfect recipe for raising stress levels and disrupting hormones. The net result is that you become less able to deal with challenging situations. Don't fall into the trap.

In the business world, companies that spend money to improve employees' health, rather than providing only traditional benefits for screening and treatment for disease, have measured return on their investment in wellness. They have found that $1 spent on keeping employees in good health returns, on average, $3. In the short term, these financial benefits accrue chiefly from a combination of fewer sick days and increased productivity and in the longer term, from significantly less high-cost medical care.

While there may be no way to precisely quantify your personal return on investment in healthier food, it requires only a little imagination to foresee consequences. Eating more unhealthy food during a stressful period may not immediately result in a life-threatening condition, but it can be debilitating. Lower levels of energy, or more pronounced fatigue and a bit of foggy thinking can seriously impact your stamina and judgment.

Sometimes, a stressful event sets off a chain reaction that throws hormones out of balance to a devastating degree. Using money to get yourself into the best possible state of health is a form of insurance, enabling you to deal with financial challenges from a position of strength.

PHYSICAL ACTIVITY

Regular exercise is a requirement for hormonal balance and overall well-being, but too much, too little or the wrong type of activity can become counterproductive by inducing stress. As a rule of thumb, forcing yourself to perform exercise you hate will promote stress, whereas doing activities you enjoy will have a relaxing effect, even if the activity is strenuous. The same activity can be stress-inducing for one person and stress-reducing for another. And, just because a certain exercise routine has worked for you in the past, don't assume it always will. Repeating the same old workout doesn't challenge muscles and produces fewer results over time. And, because of natural changes in hormone levels, your body may require a different type of approach from time to time.

Adrenal fatigue can develop from various exercise errors, including continually pushing your body beyond its capability, being very active while getting insufficient nutrients, a combination of life stress and exercise that is too intense for your own tolerance, exercising for overly long periods or giving your body insufficient time to recover between bouts of exercise. Feeling exceptionally tired the day after a workout, or even two days after a workout, is a telltale sign that your adrenals are being overtaxed, and something needs to change.

This isn't to say that you shouldn't exert yourself while exercising. Ultimately, you can't improve your fitness level without doing so. However, there are two extremes, overdoing exercise or doing none, and both work to disrupt hormones. Somewhere in between, there's an optimum level and type of activity that will lower your stress levels, stabilize your hormones, improve your mood, increase energy during the day, help you sleep well and make you feel a whole lot better. The trick is to strike that balance, to find what works for you at this particular stage of your life.

Gentle forms of exercise can help in all the above situations. These include yoga, tai chi and classes that focus on stretching, flexibility and balance. If you work hard in the gym for at least an hour every day, it may be a good idea to spend some of that time with a more soothing type of movement, such as the exercises below. If you haven't exercised for a long time, not due to any medical condition but because you hate the idea, feel too exhausted to try or simply can't find the time, these same exercises can help you get started.

LEARNING TO BREATHE

Many of us never breathe to our full capacity, shortchanging ourselves of oxygen. Taking a few deep breaths in any stressful situation can provide some immediate relief. Start by teaching yourself how to breathe right: Lie down on the floor, or the bed if that's more comfortable, and relax. Rest your hands on your stomach, fingertips touching. Take a deep breath all the way into your lungs. Your stomach should rise, pulling your fingertips apart, and your chest and shoulders should stay relaxed. Once you get used to breathing this way, you can do it sitting or standing, any time you need to relax. Taking a few deep breaths is also a good way to start your day and to relax just before going to bed.

EXERCISES FOR STRESS RELIEF

For more ways to relieve stress and tension at any time during the day, do one or more of these exercises, developed by Ivy Larson, a certified American College of Sports Medicine Health Fitness Instructor and author of several health books, including *The Gold Coast Cure*. You can feel better in a minute or so.

- While sitting, put your chest on your knees and let your head hang for 15 to 30 seconds. Feel your neck stretch out and relax.
- While standing, raise your right arm straight up and reach as high as you can while sucking in your stomach, then do the same with your left arm. Do this a few times on each side.
- Stand near a wall with your right arm extended to your side, parallel to the floor, and your right palm flat against the wall. Your arm and body should be at 90 degrees to the wall. Without moving your arm, turn your body slightly to the left. You should feel a stretch along the front of your right arm, shoulder and chest. Hold for a few seconds and repeat on the left. Do this a few times on each side.
- Stand or sit up straight and let your head slowly drop toward your chest. Roll it gently to the right, hold for a few seconds, then roll it back down and to the left and hold for a few seconds. Roll your head slowly from side to side a few more times.
- To stretch your hamstrings, stand with your right leg straight and the left knee slightly bent. Bend from the hips with a straight back, feeling a stretch on the back of your right leg. Hold a few moments and repeat on the other side. Do this a few times on each side.

A GENTLE MORNING MUSTER

Helping your body to wake up properly in the morning will put you in a better position to deal with whatever the day brings. Cheryl Patella, MS and president of Total Conditioning in Miami, developed the exercises below to gently stretch major muscles and get circulation going. When you improve blood flow, oxygen and nutrients are delivered more efficiently to all your organs and muscles, your body feels and works better and you can function with less physical stress. This routine works well if done before and after a short morning walk, or by itself.

Stay relaxed while doing these movements; they should feel good, not forced. If the floor is too uncomfortable, you can do them on the bed.

- Lie flat on the floor, hands by your sides. Relax and breathe naturally. Pull your knees into your chest, put your hands just below your knees and gently pull your thighs toward the chest. Don't let your shoulders become rounded; keep them on the floor. Feel the stretch through your back and hip joints and hold it for a few seconds, breathing normally.
- With your hands still on your knees, "walk" one knee toward you and the other one outward to a 90-degree angle to the floor, and then switch knees. Alternate sides for a total of five "walks" on each side.
- Lie flat on the floor with your knees bent and arms by your sides. Keeping your arms straight, lift them up and over your head, and then down to the floor until your hands touch the floor behind your head. Keep your body relaxed and aligned. If your shoulders are too tight to let your arms go all the way down, let them go as far

as possible or hold cans of soup to help the muscles stretch. Hold that position for 10 seconds, breathing naturally, and then return to the starting point. Repeat two more times.

- Sit up on the floor in an L shape, legs straight out in front and arms by your sides. Inhale as you lift your arms straight up above your head, then exhale as you reach toward your toes. Stay there for a few seconds, breathing normally.

- Sit up and straddle your legs in a V shape. Lean forward and try to get your elbows, bent, on the ground. If that's too difficult, get your hands on the floor in front of you, as far out as you can, and hold for a few seconds. Return to the starting position and repeat two or three times.

- Still in a straddle position, sitting up, gently rotate your torso to the right and extend your chest over your right thigh. Staying in the stretched position, swoop slowly in an arc, over to the left, so that your chest is over the left thigh, then sit up. Rotate your torso gently to the left and repeat the motion in the other direction. Repeat in both directions four more times.

- Stand up. With your weight mostly on your left leg, roll your right foot onto the toe, then back to a flat foot. Repeat a few times. Then, with only the ball of your right foot on the floor, make a circle with your knee without moving your foot. Circle to the right, then to the left, a few times in each direction. Change feet and repeat.

Research has found that reducing stress and improving well-being are more motivating reasons for exercise, among middle-age women, than weight loss. The exercises above, while not a substitute for aerobic and strength training discussed in chapter 8, should help you feel a bit better right away.

MANAGING YOUR LIFE

Recognizing that we need to do things differently as hormone levels change doesn't mean we have to "take it easy," and passively age, but it does mean we should take steps to be in the best shape possible. Managing our lives to reduce stress is something earlier generations didn't worry about, partially because they did not live as long—and when they did, they weren't faced with the challenges of a frenzied, multitasking, workaholic world.

Stress is a normal part of life, but it needs to be managed so that we can respond to emergencies or tough challenges when we need to, rather than living in a crisis situation all the time. To reduce stress levels, these are the key things to do:

- When dealing with people who create stressful situations, use a "wet towel" approach and set boundaries.
- Choose friends who bring happiness into your life.
- Include time for yourself in your daily schedule and do something you enjoy.
- Strip your to-do list of extraneous tasks.
- Use money wisely to achieve and maintain well-being.
- Learn to breathe.
- Do some gentle exercises.

7

TOXINS: REDUCING
DAILY EXPOSURE

Chemicals in our environment are complex and pervasive, and it's quite possible to become overwhelmed and stressed just by thinking about them, especially if you haven't routinely paid much attention to the subject. However, if you focus on everyday sources of toxins and replace frequently used items with non-toxic versions, it's realistic to decrease your toxic exposure without becoming obsessed with the topic.

Hormones are disrupted by chemicals we ingest in our food, absorb through our largest organ, the skin, and breathe in through our respiratory system. We can't control the outdoor air, but we certainly can reduce our exposure to toxins from conventionally grown food and synthetic food additives, beauty and grooming products, household cleaners and other products that pollute our indoor air.

Some toxins can mimic the action of hormones, such as estrogen and thyroid hormone, preventing our bodies from being able to use our own hormones and disrupting balance. In addition, toxic chemicals accumulate in tissues of glands and interfere with our ability to make hormones. Because insulin, cortisol, thyroid, estrogen, progesterone and testosterone work in concert, they are all vulnerable, directly or indirectly, to disruption by toxins. Studies have shown that common toxins in our daily lives promote early puberty and impair fertility and are linked to breast, testicular and prostate cancers, polycystic ovarian syndrome, uterine fibroids, endometriosis, miscarriage and genital birth defects in males.

Bleak as this may sound, it's possible to significantly reduce daily exposure by switching to non-toxic foods and products we use to look good and make our homes clean and fresh. Organic food is much more readily available than it was in the past, and there has been an enormous increase in the number of beauty and household products made with ingredients that don't hurt us. By taking a sensible approach, you can decrease the hormone disruptors in your environment and feel better.

FOOD

Pesticides sprayed on crops land on our plates, but the toxic burden of these drops very quickly if we switch to organic food. In a study of children, when organic foods replaced most conventionally grown ones in their diets for five days, blood levels of key pesticides were reduced to non-detectable levels. Writing in *Environmental Health Perspectives*, the researchers concluded: "An organic diet provides a dramatic and immediate protective effect."

In practice, it isn't always possible to buy organic, so it helps to set some priorities. The Environmental Working Group, a nonprofit group of scientists, identified 12 plant foods with the highest levels of pesticides, making it particularly important to buy organic versions of these:

Peaches	Apples	Sweet bell peppers
Celery	Nectarines	Strawberries

| Cherries | Lettuce | Imported grapes |
| Pears | Spinach | Potatoes |

Organic foods also contain more nutrients. This point is disputed by the food industry, perhaps because organic food makes up only a small portion of our food supply, but a considerable amount of research supports the premise. A review of nearly 100 studies found that, on average, organic fruits, vegetables and grains are 25 percent more nutritious than conventionally grown ones. Another review, which examined 41 studies, estimated that, compared to conventional crops, organic ones contain an average of 27 percent more vitamin C, 21 percent more iron, 29 percent more magnesium, 14 percent more phosphorus, lower levels of nitrates and higher-quality protein.

Conventional crops are bred to grow faster and larger than organic ones, but at a price. Faster growth seems to reduce the amount of nutrients a plant takes up from the soil and increases the amount of water content, creating bulk without nutritional substance. Organic crops grow more slowly and reach a smaller size but are more nutrient dense.

Within the American Dietetic Association, the Hunger and Environmental Nutrition Dietetic Practice Group found that organically cultivated plants tend to be richer in antioxidants than their conventional counterparts. Because they aren't sprayed with chemical pesticides, organic plants must fight harder to fend off pests, and in the process, they produce more antioxidants. And, studies that compared the flavors of strawberries and apples, grown organically and conventionally, found that organic versions had better flavor.

Meat and milk pose additional toxic challenges. When shopping, these are some things to keep in mind.

- Meat from conventionally raised cows contains several toxins: pesticide residue from the feed of the animals, growth hormones given to the cows to increase their size, and antibiotics used to ward off disease among animals raised in cramped quarters. The hormones can impact our own hormones, and the antibiotics contribute to antibiotic resistance.
- The use of the same types of growth enhancers in chickens has decreased somewhat and varies from one brand to another.
- Growth hormone isn't generally used in raising pigs, but antibiotics may be given to the animals.
- Toxins accumulate mostly in the fat of animals, so fatty cuts contain the most toxins.
- Organic milk, meat and poultry come from animals raised without growth promoters or pesticides in their feed, and are a much healthier choice.

On food labels, the word "organic" doesn't necessarily mean that everything in a packaged food is organic. However, the use of the term is regulated, and products or ingredients that are certified organic must be produced according to set criteria, including these:

- Crops must be grown without the use of synthetic herbicides and pesticides, genetic modification, irradiation or the use of processed sewage sludge.

- Organic farm land must be free of chemical application for at least three years.
- Livestock must eat organically grown feed without any animal byproducts, must have access to pasture and cannot be given growth hormone or antibiotics.

These are the basic ways "organic" may appear on labels of packaged foods:

PRODUCT LABEL	PROPORTION OF CERTIFIED ORGANIC INGREDIENTS
100% organic	100%
Organic	95%
Made with organic ingredients	70%
When one or more ingredients are organic but make up less than 70%, "organic" can only be used to describe the ingredient on the ingredient list, not on the overall product label.	

The term "natural" appears on many food labels, but it isn't regulated. The U.S. Department of Agriculture has established that natural meat and poultry should contain no artificial flavor, color, chemical preservative or any other synthetic ingredient and that it should be "minimally processed," but there is no definition of minimal processing. Because the criteria for a "natural" label do not prevent an animal from being raised with growth hormone and antibiotics, the contents of natural meat and poultry vary. Unless the packaging contains a full explanation, it's wise to ask someone at the meat counter about the practices of the store's suppliers.

Food additives in packaged foods and beverages can cause adverse reactions and contribute to disruption of normal hormonal function. MSG (monosodium glutamate) is considered safe by the government, but some people experience adverse reactions from the flavor enhancer, including headaches, numbness, tingling, a burning sensation, chest pain, drowsiness, nausea, a faster heart beat and weight gain. On labels, MSG may be listed as glutamate, glutamic acid, or may be in other ingredients, such as yeast extract, textured protein, gelatin, calcium caseinate, sodium caseinate or flavoring. Other ingredients, used to add flavor or color, or to preserve food, can also cause problems.

Fish present another problem: mercury and other pollutants found in oceans, rivers and lakes. Safe choices include wild salmon, canned salmon, farmed rainbow trout, sardines, and farmed and wild shrimp from North America. The Environmental Defense Fund (www.edf.org) provides updated information on many types of fish and seafood.

The process of trying to weed out toxins from your food could get complex enough to become another source of stress, which would be counterproductive. The main thing to be aware of is that minimizing toxins in your food is a basic way to protect your hormones from disruption and to improve your state of health.

Don't become obsessed with the subject but do aim to buy organic versions of the staples in your diet as much as possible or choose the most wholesome versions you can find, such as lean beef raised without growth hormones. For packaged foods, remember this one simple rule: The longer the list of ingredients that aren't found in nature, the more likely it is that the product may contribute to hormonal imbalance.

WATER

Bottled water has become a controversial subject because tests of some products have revealed that they contain tap water, and other tests have found higher levels of bacteria in some bottled water than in tap water. If you buy bottled spring water, you may want to check on the practices of the company whose products you buy.

Filtered water is another alternative, especially if you install a high-quality filtration system for your entire house, giving you safer water for drinking, cooking and bathing. Another option is installing one filter on your kitchen tap and another on your showerhead. Many types of filters are available, and it's a wise move to buy the best quality you can afford.

PLASTICS

The idea that all contact between plastic and food is dangerous can easily throw you into panic mode, but fortunately, this doesn't seem to be the case. However, plastic should not be heated. Heat can trigger release of chemicals, even from microwave-safe containers, which are safe from the standpoint of not disintegrating but otherwise, there are no assurances. It's best to use microwave-safe ceramic or glass containers. Even without heat, some plastics can leach chemicals such as phthalates, described below.

Plastic storage containers are made with different types of resins, and are marked accordingly. If you flip a plastic container upside down, there is usually a triangle with a number on the bottom, indicating the resin type. Containers marked #2, 4 or 5 are designed to be re-used and do not leach chemicals. Those marked #1 are for one-time use and should not be re-used but otherwise, they are safe. However, containers marked #3, 6 or 7 can leach chemicals and should be avoided.

Plastics made from corn, potatoes or other plants are another safe and environmentally sustainable option, when available. Plastic wrap and freezer and sandwich bags may or may not leach chemicals, depending on the brand. The Green Guide (www.thegreenguide.com) of the National Geographic Society provides updated lists of specific safe brands, which include Glad Wrap and Ziploc freezer and sandwich bags.

BISPHENOL A (BPA) IN PLASTICS AND CANS

BPA is used in making plastic products and to line the insides of cans. The chemical leaches from plastic containers marked #7, which have been used in some baby bottles and some re-usable water bottles, and from those marked #3 or 6. When used as a lining for cans, BPA may leach into food, especially if the contents of a can are acidic, such as tomatoes, fruit juices and soda.

In the human body, BPA mimics estrogen, which contributes to unhealthy, elevated levels of the hormone and disrupts balance with progesterone and testosterone. In fetuses and infants, BPA may harm the brain and prostate. Some cans and plastic products are BPA-free, and state so on product packaging. It's wise to steer clear of BPA.

FRAGRANCE

We are exposed to synthetic scents from different sources, including air fresheners, scented candles, laundry and dishwashing detergents, household cleaners, and beauty and grooming products. Fragrance formulas are regarded as trade secrets, and there is no legal requirement for manufacturers to disclose ingredients in their scents or to prove that they are safe. Consequently, "fragrance" or "scent" on a product label usually means synthetic scents that contain toxins such as phthalates and/or parabens.

PHTHALATES

Pronounced "tha-layts" (rhymes with "waits"), these chemicals reduce levels of sex hormones and contribute to poor sperm quality, infertility, genital birth defects and possibly cancer. Phthalates are used to soften vinyl plastics, which would otherwise be brittle, and can leach from unsafe types of plastic food containers (#3, 6 or 7). They are found in some toys, give new vinyl shower curtains their distinct odor and may be partially responsible for "new car smell." Unless a specific product clearly states something to the contrary, "scent" or "fragrance" generally indicates the presence of phthalates. These toxins are a component of fragrance in a wide range of products including many skin creams and lotions, cosmetics, soaps, cleansers, face and body scrubs, shampoos, conditioners, and home cleaning, laundry and air freshening products. Phthalates are also found in nail polishes and treatments.

PARABENS

A class of chemical preservatives used to kill bacteria in water-based products, parabens may be a component of fragrance or a separate ingredient in beauty products, including liquid soaps, lotions, cleansers, facial and body scrubs, shampoos and hair conditioners. When they occur only in fragrance, parabens will not be listed as an ingredient on product labels. There is some controversy as to the degree of danger they pose, but parabens have been linked to hormone disruption, skin irritation and cancer.

ANTIBACTERIAL PRODUCTS

Many soaps, wipes, hand sanitizers, dish soaps and other cleansers are promoted for their antibacterial action, but this may be a liability rather than an asset. Despite the wide promotion of bug-killing cleansers, they don't appear to be any more effective than ordinary soaps in protecting us against infection. Traditional soaps work by making it easier for dirt and germs to slide off skin, but antibacterial ingredients go a step further and kill bugs. Antibacterial ingredients have become so prevalent that they have created superbugs that are resistant to antibiotics and other medications used to treat serious illness. And, there's a toxic side to at least one germ killer, triclosan.

TRICLOSAN

A widely used antibacterial (also referred to as antimicrobial) ingredient, triclosan is found in toothpaste, dishwashing liquid, deodorants, soaps, some antibacterial creams, detergents, fabrics with an antibacterial or antimicrobial claim and other products. Technically, triclosan is a pesticide, and, according to animal research, it disrupts the function of thyroid hormone and is potentially carcinogenic. When mixed with warm water at a temperature typically used in the home (100 degrees Fahrenheit or higher), triclosan rapidly degrades into chloroform, a toxic chemical, but the degree to which this phenomena may harm human health is a controversial topic. Proponents of triclosan say alarm is unwarranted, but it's wise to stay away from this and other antibacterial ingredients in all types of cleansers. Coming into contact with a surface cleaned with an antibacterial substance, as well as using antibacterial soaps, creams or lotions, are ways to ingest triclosan.

TOXIN REDUCTION BASICS

While this chapter doesn't cover every possible source of toxicity, it does address some key sources that we can control on a daily basis. Toxins are a significant contributor to any type of hormonal imbalance but reducing our exposure can be confusing and stressful. To keep things simple, first try the A-list below, and then give yourself more anti-toxin support as you progress.

THE ANTI-TOXIN A-LIST

- Keep your home well ventilated and eliminate sources of unpleasant odors rather than masking them with air fresheners that contain synthetic fragrances. To "freshen" your house, open doors and windows. In extreme weather, use common sense and keep in mind that toxins in an insulated, sealed building will linger for longer periods of time.
- Choose organic food and milk whenever possible.
- Drink filtered water.
- Avoid synthetic fragrance and antibacterial ingredients in beauty, grooming and household products.

MORE ANTI-TOXIN SUPPORT

- To choose healthier grooming and beauty products, check ingredients and potential toxic hazards of specific brands in the Skin Deep Cosmetic Safety Database, created by the Environmental Working Group at www.cosmetic database.com. The largest database of its kind, it contains toxicity information on more than 41,000 products.

- When heating food in the microwave, use microwave-safe ceramic or glass containers rather than plastic ones.

- When using plastic containers for food storage or beverages, choose those marked #2, 4 or 5 on the bottom, and don't heat them. For safe plastic product brands, check the National Geographic Society's Green Guide at www.thegreenguide.com.

- When buying beverages in plastic bottles designed for one-time use, check the number on the bottom of the container; it should be #1.

- When buying canned food, look for BPA-free cans. Otherwise, buy acidic foods and beverages, such as sodas, fruit juices and tomato sauces, in bottles, jars or cartons instead of cans.

- When buying household cleaners, look for ones that are biodegradable, plant-based, enzyme-based, chlorine-free or phosphate-free, and don't contain synthetic fragrance. Products that are good for the environment tend to be pretty safe for humans.

8

EXERCISE FOR HARMONY

When was the last time someone told you they regretted being fit? In contrast, how often do hear: "I know I should get some exercise but ..."? The latter sentiment is understandable, even forgivable, but not unchangeable.

Physical activity is the closest thing we have to the proverbial fountain of youth, but the tangible benefits can be difficult to imagine until you experience them. If you aren't already a fan of exercise, getting started can be the biggest obstacle. However, when it comes to hormonal harmony, exercise is directly related.

Physical activity plays a key role in reversing insulin resistance, the phenomenon that triggers hormonal imbalance. This is how it works: Remember that insulin resistance occurs after muscle cells are repeatedly bombarded with too much fuel, in the form of blood sugar, because of a diet that is too rich in sugary, starchy carbohydrates. Those muscle cells have literally closed their doors, and consequently, fuel gets diverted to fat cells. However, with the right exercise, the body builds new muscles cells. Those virgin cells are especially valuable because, in effect, they didn't get the memo about closing their doors, so they gladly accept fuel. At the same time, exercise helps old muscle cells to wake up to the fact that they need some fuel, so they begin to reopen their doors.

In a nutshell, that's how exercise can help to reverse the whole insidious cycle of insulin resistance, turning off the switch that disrupts hormones. To reap the full benefits, you need strength training for your muscles and aerobic exercise for your heart. If you're inactive and over 40, or have a medical condition, get your doctor's approval before beginning a fitness program.

TAKING CARE OF MUSCLES

Call it a cruel trick of nature if you like, but the longer we live, the less muscle we possess. After the age of 30, people who are physically inactive lose anywhere from 3 to 5 percent of their total muscle mass per decade. After age 50, without adequate strength training, the rate of muscle loss can double, translating into an average loss of 5 pounds of muscle per decade for women and 7 pounds per decade for men. This phenomenon is the biggest reason why elderly people become frail, and it is a basic cause of weight gain that seems to be a "normal" part of aging.

Losing muscle means losing strength, making any type of physical exertion more taxing and less appealing, and it breeds more inactivity. As the amount of muscle declines, a body needs less fuel in the form of food. Consequently, even if you don't eat more as you live longer, more and more of your food calories will be stored as fat, unless you do something to counteract muscle shrinkage. And with age, our bodies become less efficient at converting the protein we eat into muscle tissue, adding impetus to the muscle-wasting process.

There's a technical term for this unwelcome, age-related loss of muscle mass and strength: sarcopenia (pronounced "sarkopean-ya"), derived from the Greek words for "loss of flesh." The condition is a huge problem for elderly people who become frail to the point of not being able to get out of a chair or walk across a room without assistance. This degree of frailty doesn't develop overnight, but surprisingly, it can be reversed to a great degree— and quite quickly—with strength training. Studies of nursing home residents have found that as little as two weeks of strength-building exercises, with weights or some other type of resistance, can produce dramatic changes in people's ability to function.

Long before frailty is an issue, the symptoms of muscle loss are much more subtle and insidious. Perhaps the scale says you haven't gained weight, but your clothes aren't as comfortable, or you just don't feel as good in a bathing suit. Or, as is often the case, extra pounds visibly creep on and refuse to budge, helping to disrupt hormones and increasing risk for chronic disease and disability.

STRENGTH-TRAINING BASICS

There's no substitute for strength training. Leading fitness expert Wayne Wescott, Ph.D., fitness research director for the South Shore YMCA in Quincy, Massachusetts, author of 20 books on exercise and a fitness consultant for major government and private organizations, puts it this way: "If you only do aerobic exercise as you progress through the aging process, you will still lose muscle mass and you will still reduce your resting metabolic rate almost as much as if you were doing no exercise at all."

On the bright side, it doesn't take a tremendous amount of time and effort to reverse the metabolic decline. Wescott tested

IMPORTANT REASONS TO EXERCISE

Be Happy

Exercise triggers production of endorphins, feel-good chemicals. And, research shows that it both prevents and alleviates depression at any age. For women approaching or going through menopause, it also stabilizes mood swings.

Keep Blood Sugar Stable

By helping to stabilize blood-sugar levels, exercise counteracts spikes and crashes that trigger hormonal imbalance.

Control Your Weight

Statistically, the most likely way to achieve and maintain a healthy weight is by combining exercise with a healthy diet.

Control Your Appetite

Exercise, especially aerobic activity, suppresses appetite by acting on hormones that regulate hunger.

Live Longer

Both men and women gain healthy years with regular exercise.

Keep Bones Strong

At any age, regular exercise improves bone density, which is especially important for preventing osteoporosis after menopause.

Prevent Cancers

Exercise helps to prevent breast and ovarian cancers, slows progression of prostate cancer, and reduces risk for colorectal cancers in both men and women.

Protect Vision

Vigorous exercise reduces the risks of cataracts and age-related macular degeneration, two leading causes of vision loss.

Improve Joint Function

Exercise reduces the likelihood of arthritis and where the condition already exists, helps to reduce pain and improve joint function.

Be Good to Your Heart

For men and women who exercise, the chance of suffering a heart attack or death from heart disease is only a fraction of the risk faced by their sedentary peers.

Reduce Risk of Stroke

Fit people have somewhere between one-third and one-half the risk of a stroke, compared to those who are unfit.

Maintain a Healthy Brain

Overall fitness keeps the brain in good shape and reduces risk for Alzheimer's disease and other types of dementia.

Prevent Diabetes

Any type of regular exercise, such as walking, reduces risk for type 2 diabetes. More vigorous activity reduces risk to a greater degree.

Avoid Incontinence

For women, walking and other types of exercise reduce the chances of developing incontinence.

a basic 10-week exercise program on 1,644 mostly sedentary people between the ages of 21 and 80 and found that at least two weekly gym sessions, each consisting of 20 minutes of aerobics and 20 minutes of strength training, significantly improved body composition.

The study compared the effects of two and three workouts per week, and found that in a 10-week program, three weekly workouts produced more fat loss: 4.4 pounds compared to 3.2 pounds for two weekly workouts. However, both programs added the same amount of muscle, an average of 3.1 pounds.

How significant are these changes? "Other research has shown that three pounds of strength-training muscle will increase your resting metabolic rate by 7 percent," says Wescott, "which reverses about 14 years of the aging process."

In terms of basic biology, science also shows that strength training improves the body's ability to utilize protein to sustain and increase muscle tissue. And, it improves internal production of hormones that decline with age.

To start improving your body composition, Wescott recommends:

COVER THE BASICS. Do at least 20 minutes of aerobic exercise three times per week, and strength training twice per week, working all your major muscle groups. For each resistance exercise, do 8 to 12 repetitions (one "set" in fitness terms) with a weight that leaves you fatigued at the end of the set. Increase weight in increments of about 5 percent as you become stronger. As you progress, you can add a second, and then a third set for each exercise.

DON'T MAKE "NO TIME" AN EXCUSE. You can get tangible results in two weekly workouts, at home or at a health club, each including a combination of aerobic and strength training that takes less than an hour. A third aerobic session could be done at home, at a health club, or on a weekend hike, bike ride or other fun excursion, such as an evening of dancing.

There are many books and videos with various strength-training routines, but the best way to learn proper form and technique is to work with a personal trainer, at least until you get the hang of it. For a sample workout, see *A Basic Strength-Training Routine* at the end of this chapter.

AEROBIC EXERCISE

Regular aerobic exercise literally slows down the aging process. It improves the body's ability to take in and use oxygen to generate energy, a process that begins to deteriorate in middle age but can be reversed. Biologically speaking, some researchers have estimated that aerobic exercise can make a body function as though it were 12 years younger, as well as preventing major diseases and speeding recovery from illness and injury.

The heart is the most important muscle in our bodies, and aerobic exercise strengthens it and keeps it pumping at its best. To accomplish this, it's necessary to get the heart to exert itself a bit more, meaning beat faster, than it does in the normal course of a day. How much faster and for how long depends on what you're trying to accomplish. An athlete training for an Olympic sprint has different training needs than someone who wants to stay healthy and fit and keep their hormones in optimum balance.

For hormonal harmony, there are two main objectives: To reduce body fat or maintain it at healthy levels and to keep the heart healthy. In numerical terms, the intensity of aerobic exercise is measured by heart rate—the number of times the heart beats in a minute. For aerobic benefits, the main point is to do some activity vigorously enough to make the heart beat faster than it normally does in the course of the day—to elevate the heart rate.

In Wescott's study, which concurs with the overall body of research on the subject, aerobic exercise was done at 70 percent of maximum heart rate. The important thing is to establish what that means for you, which depends mostly on your fitness level.

If you want to look at this very simply, without any math, let's say you're walking. Aim to walk briskly enough to breathe more heavily than usual but still be able to talk. However, if you can easily sing your favorite song, pick up the pace.

If you want to be more precise, which is not a bad idea, try one of these methods to figure out 70 percent of your maximum heart rate.

- Go to a health club or sports medicine clinic and ask to get tested to determine your maximum heart rate, and then multiply that number by 0.7. You will pay a fee and get an accurate number.
- Walk really fast or run until you're heart is beating so fast, you simply can't go any faster. (Make sure your doctor doesn't object before you do this.) Take your pulse on the side of your neck while looking at the

second hand of a watch to get your maximum heart rate, and multiply it by 0.7 to get 70 percent. Without math, consider that peak of exertion to be a 10 on a scale of 1 to 10, estimate what 7 would feel like and aim for that pace.

- As a rough guide, subtract your age from 220, then multiply that number by 0.7, which will give you 70 percent of your maximum heart rate. For example, this is the calculation if your are 50 years old:

$$220 - 50 = 170 \text{ X } 0.7 = 119$$

In the above example, 119 would be the number of beats per minute to aim for in your aerobic exercise. To check your approximate heart rate per minute, you can take your pulse for 6 seconds and multiply by 10. For example, if your heart beats 12 times in 6 seconds, your heart rate (12 X 10) is 120 beats per minute, which is close enough to the target 119. Or, you can take your pulse for 10 seconds, which may be a bit more accurate, and multiply by 6. In this example, 20 beats in 10 seconds (20 X 6) would be 120 beats per minute. (To be mathematically precise, 19.83 beats in 10 seconds equates to 119 beats per minute but it's physically impossible to take your pulse with that degree of accuracy.) Because individual fitness levels vary at any age, keep in mind that this is an estimate. If you feel as though you're exercising at a level that is too difficult or too easy, go with what feels right to you.

MONITORING HEART RATE

Wearing a heart rate monitor is the most accurate way to track your heart rate, and while it may seem like a bother to even think about a gadget, it's a valuable tool. Some people find that heart rate monitors are motivating, and they can definitely help you to get the most out of your aerobic exercise time. On the other hand, if the thought of dealing with a gadget makes you less likely to exercise, skip it.

If you want to consider a heart rate monitor, be aware that they are available in these two varieties:

- The most accurate type consists of a sensor on a strap that goes around your chest, underneath your clothes, and a monitor, on a wrist strap, which looks like a watch. The sensor tracks your heart beat and transmits the number of beats per minute to the wrist component, and your heart rate appears continuously on what looks like the face of a watch on your wrist. The simplest and least expensive models display only your heart rate, but some also function as a watch. More complex and costly versions store data and enable it to be uploaded to your computer and, in some cases, a web site to track your workouts. If you like tracking progress with numbers, you might find it motivating to track your workout statistics.

- The other type of heart rate monitor consists only of a wrist component like a watch, which may also function as a watch. It's easier to wear but not as efficient because you have to touch a sensor with a finger whenever you want to measure and see your heart rate. You have to interrupt your motion, if only briefly, to check your heart rate, so this system is less accurate and can be a distraction. However, if you find that it helps you to get fit, it's a good gadget.

Heart rate monitoring is useful to help you stay in your optimum range and get a good aerobic workout without overdoing it. If you experience hot flashes while doing aerobic exercise, you'll probably have to slow down to maintain your optimum heart rate, which is good from the standpoint of safety and comfort.

A fit heart pumps more blood with each beat than a heart that is out of shape, so the fit heart doesn't have to work as hard at any level of activity. In numerical terms, a fit person can do more vigorous exercise with a lower heart rate, whereas the heart rate of an unfit person will increase much more with only a slight increase in effort. As you become more fit, you will have to work more intensely to reach your target heart rate, which means you're constantly improving your physical state. Monitoring heart rate is a good way to make sure you push yourself a bit, but not too much, and increase your aerobic intensity and cardiovascular fitness at a safe pace.

DO YOU NEED A HEALTH CLUB?

Exercising at home is a very popular option, and it doesn't require purchasing expensive equipment. In addition to sticking with your own commitment to yourself, it helps if you designate a space where you won't be distracted. If you use an exercise DVD, try to arrange things so that no one disturbs your workout. If you're doing strength training, it's ideal if you can see yourself in a mirror, such as a full-length closet mirror, to make sure your posture and form are maintained. The most important thing is to be in your exercise space and not allow others to interfere during your time.

A lot of people are intimidated by health clubs, but the stereotype of a gym full of iron-pumping, muscle-bound men is history. While there are gyms that cater specifically to male and female body builders, most health clubs are experiencing their largest growth among baby boomers and older people.

The best way to decide if a health club might be right for you is to check out different ones in your area. Get a tour of each club and find out about personal training as well as classes. Most likely, the tour will end with a sales pitch but don't be intimidated. Rather than getting into a discussion or trying to get a salesperson to agree with you (it's their job to disagree with anything but your signature on the dotted line), just say, "No, thank you," unless you really want to join. Better yet, ask if free passes are available to try out a club, take advantage of any offers and get a sense of whether the place is right for you. If sales people intimidate you, ask a friend to come along for the tour. And check out local community centers, as many of these offer a variety of interesting fitness classes.

MAKING TIME

For overall health, most people who live a typical Western lifestyle will reap significant health benefits from walking for 30 minutes a day, either nonstop or in shorter segments spread throughout the day. For weight loss, walking an hour a day is more likely to produce results. The alternative is to exercise more intensely for shorter periods, as in the study described above.

If you suffer from debilitating joint pain or have other physical limitations, it's a matter of finding the right type of exercise and then fitting it into your schedule. Many community centers and health clubs have classes tailored for people with joint problems. Most often, these are done in a pool so that water supports body weight to avoid stress on joints. With even a little weight loss and increased muscle strength, joints function better, and you may soon be able to progress to other types of activities. In some situations, it's easier to start with strength training and add aerobic exercise at a later stage. If you have a physical condition that limits your movement, physicians or physical therapists can help you find the appropriate type of exercise program.

The key thing is to build activity into your life. The process starts with putting exercise on your daily list of tasks that simply must be done, just like brushing your teeth, and setting realistic goals. For example, if you haven't done any exercise for a long time and are overweight, start by walking down the street as far as you can. It doesn't matter if it's halfway down the block. On each of the next few days, walk the same distance until it seems comfortable, and then go a little farther. When starting out, the most common mistake is to do too much, too quickly, experience a setback and give up. If you are consistent and allow yourself to progress at a slow but steady pace, you'll be amazed at how much your fitness can improve in a relatively short period of time.

A BASIC STRENGTH-TRAINING ROUTINE

Do 8 to 12 repetitions of each exercise with a weight that leaves you fatigued at the end of the set. When working each arm or leg separately, do 8 to 12 repetitions with each one. Aim to take about six seconds to complete each repetition. If you find squats or lunges difficult, start without weights. Allow at least one day between workouts to give muscles time to recover. Sporting goods stores sell dumbbells for a few dollars.

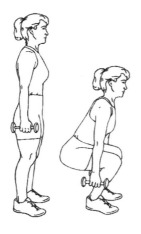

SQUAT (works thighs and buttocks) Stand with your feet shoulder-width apart. Keeping you back straight and head up, bend your knees until your thighs are parallel to floor, maintaining your weight on your heels. Keep your abdominals tight throughout the exercise. Straighten and repeat.

LUNGE (works thighs and buttocks) Stand with your feet shoulder-width apart, head up and back straight. Step forward with your right leg, bending the knee until your thigh is parallel to floor. Keep the front knee over the foot, not in front of it. Return to the starting position. Repeat with the left leg and continue to alternate legs.

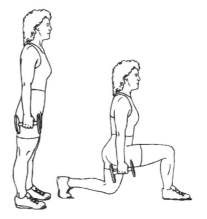

SIDE BEND (works abdominals)

Tighten your abdominals and bend to one side as far as possible without straining, return to the starting position. Do a set on one side, then on the other side.

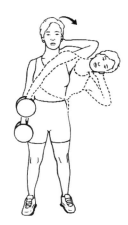

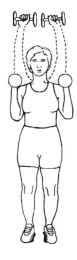

SHOULDER PRESS (works shoulders)

Stand with your knees slightly bent, palms facing inward. Press up to straight arms, rotating your palms to face forward at end of movement. Return to the starting position.

BENT ROW (works the back)

Stand on your right leg with your left knee and hand resting on a bench (or a sturdy trunk or couch). Bend from the hips and keep the back, neck and head in a straight line, approximately parallel to the floor. Starting with

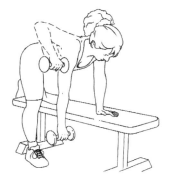

your right arm straight down, lift the weight to the side of your chest, pulling the elbow back and keeping it close to your body. Return to the staring position and repeat. When the set is complete, do a set on the other side.

BENCH PRESS (works the chest)

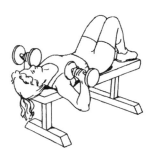 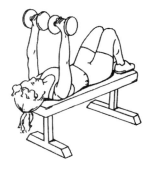 This can be done on the floor but works best on a bench by allowing the arms to drop down farther in the starting position. Press up above your chest to straighten the arms and return to the starting position.

TRICEP KICKBACK (works the back of the upper arm)

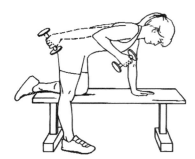 Start in the same position as the bent row but with the right elbow bent and the upper arm close in to your torso. Straighten the arm, keeping upper arm in line with your body, and return to the starting position.

BICEP CURL (works the front of the upper arm)

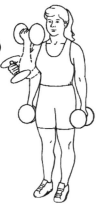 Stand with your knees slightly bent, holding the weights at your sides with your palms facing your body. Curl one arm toward shoulder, rotating it so that the palm faces you at the top of the movement. Return to the starting position and repeat with the other arm.

9

SUPPLEMENTS: THE BASICS

Dietary supplements aren't a substitute for a healthy diet, but they help to fill in dietary gaps and provide nutritional support to help meet the challenges your body faces from the environment and life's stresses. In terms of hormonal function, you can think of a good quality multivitamin, mineral and antioxidant combination as the first part of a foundation for balance. It should be accompanied with fish oil and CoQ10, which are not found in multivitamins. And, for optimum health, you will need magnesium and vitamins C and D in greater quantities than those found in multivitamins.

For a snapshot of what to look for, see the *Shopping Guide* at the end of the chapter. Supplements that can help in specific situations are covered in the next chapter.

MULTIVITAMINS

Commonly referred to as "multis," multivitamins are available in pills, powders and liquids, and the quantities and scope of nutrients they contain vary significantly. The choices can be very confusing, but they become easier to deal with if you recognize that there are basically three categories of multi formulations. Which one you choose depends on your own needs and goals. Keep in mind that the benefits come from getting these nutrients on a consistent basis.

You could consider these three categories as grades of dietary supplements.

AVAILABLE IN DRUG STORES AND SUPERMARKETS: The more traditional multis, the most popular type found in these retail stores, contain very small amounts of most essential vitamins and minerals. Some brands contain artificial flavors, preservatives and coloring dyes. You could call these low-dose multis, and they have the lowest price tag.

AVAILABLE IN HEALTH FOOD STORES, NATURAL SUPERMARKETS AND ONLINE: This category of multis contains larger amounts of essential nutrients, and some brands contain a wide range of antioxidants and other beneficial ingredients not found in the low-dose variety. This category of multis does not, as a rule, contain artificial flavors, preservatives or coloring dyes. As you might expect, their price tag is higher.

AVAILABLE FROM LICENSED HEALTH PROFESSIONALS: Some companies manufacture dietary supplements for distribution only through medical doctors and other licensed health professionals. These types of multis tend to contain an even broader range of nutrients, especially important antioxidants, and other ingredients that make it easier for a human body to utilize the whole formula. The manufacturers in this category make a greater investment in research related to their product formulations, in strictly controlling standards and purity of their products, and in educating health professionals about related science. In some cases, the price tag on these multis is much like some brands sold in health food stores and in others, the health-professional brands cost a little more. (If you're wondering where these are available in your area, see *Supplement Sources* in the Appendix.)

Which type of multi you take depends upon your personal goals. Low-dose multis are designed to prevent very basic deficiencies. If you're striving for optimum health, you'll be better served by higher-quality products with a more comprehensive range of nutrients in quantities shown to enhance overall well-being.

To support hormonal balance and good health, below are some of the key ingredients to look for in a multi. See the *Shopping Guide* chart at the end of this chapter for quantities of each nutrient.

ANTIOXIDANTS

Each antioxidant nutrient has unique qualities, and a combination offers the most protection. Beta-carotene, which gives carrots their signature color, is a precursor to vitamin A (meaning our bodies turn beta-carotene into vitamin A), and it is a fairly common ingredient in all types of multis. However, there are other nutrients in the same family, known as carotenoids, which give other plant foods their vivid colors and, collectively, contain a broader spectrum of antioxidants. More comprehensive multi formulas contain a mixture of these, most often listed on labels as "mixed

SPECIAL ANTIOXIDANT FORMULAS

The process of oxidation is what causes a sliced apple to turn brown or a pipe to rust. In our bodies, oxidation is a byproduct of normal life for which our bodies have built-in antioxidant defenses. Plant foods naturally contain antioxidants that can provide additional protection. However, poor nutrition and exposure to man-made toxins leave our bodies susceptible to oxidative damage, which has been linked with many conditions, including rheumatoid arthritis, asthma, decrease in bone density, chronic fatigue syndrome, digestive conditions, diseases of the liver, kidney and pancreas, and neurological disorders. Being overweight, physically inactive or generally being in poor health increases levels of oxidation.

Special antioxidant formulas offer extra protection with combinations of strong antioxidants that work together synergistically. Here's a list of key ingredients in such products, which can be taken in addition to a multi.

Grape Seed Extract

The seeds of grapes are the source of many benefits attributed to the fruit. In studies, grape seed extract has improved symptoms of poor circulation in the legs, reducing leg swelling and heaviness, as well as reducing swelling, pain and strange sensations (known as paresthesias) after surgery. In addition to being a strong antioxidant, the extract has been found to act as a gentle blood thinner, help to reduce blood pressure and prevent dangerous cholesterol from oxidizing, and may provide relief from allergies and asthma.

Pycnogenol

Many studies have tested a proprietary extract of pine bark known as Pycnogenol (pronounced "pick-gnaw-ju-nol"). They have found that Pycnogenol may help prevent heart disease and diabetes and provide some relief from circulatory disorders, eye conditions, PMS, menopausal symptoms, ADHD, male infertility, osteoarthritis, gum disease, asthma, hay fever, sun damage to skin, post-exercise pain and cramps. The extract has blood-thinning properties and helps to reduce the risk of blood clots on long flights.

Both grape seed extract and Pycnogenol contain a collection of nutrients that are categorized as OPCs (oligomeric proantho-cyanidin complexes); both fight bacteria, viruses and inflammation and may reduce the risk of cancer. Because each extract has a unique combination of OPCs, the two can be taken together.

Citrus Bioflavonoids

Bioflavonoids, also called flavonoids, are a group of nutrients that give plants their distinctive colors. In nature, bioflavonoids occur in fruits and vegetables that also contain vitamin C, and they enhance the benefits of the vitamin. Bioflavonoids found in citrus fruits strengthen the walls of blood vessels and improve the function of the lymph system. They may help to relieve hemorrhoids and improve the health of weak veins in the legs (chronic venous insufficiency). People who bruise easily or tend to suffer from nosebleeds may also benefit from citrus bioflavonoids. And in one study of women, these nutrients helped reduce swelling of lymph nodes in the arm after breast cancer surgery.

Quercetin

Quercetin is one of the bioflavonoids in citrus fruits, but it is also found in other foods, such as apples, parsley and onions, and in tea and red wine. In addition to being an antioxidant, quercetin fights inflammation and acts as an antihistamine. It may reduce symptoms of allergic reactions, inflammation of the prostate (prostatitis), arterial damage that contributes to heart disease and chronic inflammation of the bladder known as interstitial cystitis, and may help prevent cancer.

carotenoids." The key word to look for is "carotenoids," the plural being the important detail. Other antioxidants found in better quality multis, but not in low-dose products, may include citrus bioflavonoids or bioflavonoids, lycopene, lutein and quercetin.

VITAMIN A

Vitamin A and its building blocks, the carotenoids, support healthy eyesight, protect against heart disease and cancer, may reduce sun sensitivity and are necessary for healthy skin. Unlike carotenoids, too much vitamin A can be toxic. On the other hand, it's possible that some people don't efficiently convert carotenoids to vitamin A. A multi with both vitamin A and a mixture of carotenoids is a good option. Multi labels may list vitamin A and beta-carotene at the top of the ingredients list and mixed carotenoids separately, further down in the Supplement Facts panel.

B VITAMINS

We need adequate B vitamins for efficient conversion of carbo-hydrates into energy and to break down fats and protein. Collectively known as B complex, they include B1 (thiamine), B2 (riboflavin), B3 (niacin or niacinamide), B5 (pantothenic acid), B6 (pyridoxine), B12 (cobalamin) and folic acid (described in more detail below). The Bs support muscle tone in the digestive system and promote healthy eyes, skin, hair and liver. They are also necessary for proper function of the nervous system and are good nutritional buffers against the effects of stress. These are some other benefits of individual B vitamins: B12 may help to alleviate depression and age-related memory problems, and a deficiency of B12 contributes to anemia. A combination of B6,

B12 and folic acid reduces levels of homocysteine, which is associated with malfunction of the lining of blood vessels, a risk factor for heart disease and stroke. In a study of more than 5,000 women, the same combination, taken daily for at least two years, reduced risk for age-related macular degeneration, a leading cause of vision loss. And a preliminary study found that a combination of B vitamins, including folic acid, may reduce the frequency and intensity of migraines, although further research is needed to determine optimum amounts.

FOLIC ACID

Although it is a B vitamin (B9), folic acid merits special attention because it is added to some foods, such as some cereals, and is listed separately in all multis, even low-dose ones. The minimum quantity in all multis is usually 400 mcg because, when women routinely get this amount in the early stages of pregnancy, folic acid reduces the risk of their babies being born with brain and spinal defects. Because conception isn't always planned, it's advisable for all women of child-bearing age to take at least 400 mcg of folic acid on a regular basis. For people of all ages, folic acid is associated with reduced risk for heart disease, depression and Alzheimer's disease. Where these additional benefits have been found in studies, higher dosages have often been used. In the vision study mentioned above, women took 2,500 mcg of folic acid, along with 50 mg of B6 and 1,000 mcg of B12.

VITAMIN C

An antioxidant, vitamin C is especially important during times of life stress, when recovering from an injury or illness, and whenever physical activity is significantly increased. Even in the best of circumstances, our bodies require vitamin C for virtually every aspect of wellness, including healthy skin, heart function, protection against cancer and a healthy immune system. Low levels of the vitamin correlate with excess weight and may promote cravings for sweet or salty snacks, or beverages that are sugary or contain stimulants, such as caffeine. Because vitamin C is water soluble, any amounts we can't absorb are excreted (extreme overdose can produce diarrhea). To utilize the nutrient effectively, break down your daily intake into several doses. Bioflavonoids, nutrients found in citrus fruits, are also antioxidants and may enhance the benefits of vitamin C. Higher-quality multis often contain bioflavonoids.

VITAMIN D

As a rule, multis will not contain adequate vitamin D. Once considered to be primarily a bone-building nutrient, because it regulates calcium absorption, more recent research shows that vitamin D plays a much bigger role in overall health. Conditions linked to insufficient vitamin D include these cancers: bladder, breast, cervical, colon, endometrial, esophageal, gallbladder, gastric, Hodgkin's lymphoma, laryngeal, non-Hodgkin's lymphoma, oral, ovarian, pancreatic, prostate, rectal and renal. Other conditions linked to low levels of the vitamin include chronic low back pain, colds, type 1 diabetes, increased risk of falls and fractures, flu, heart disease, hyperparathyroidism, hypertension, melanoma, mental illness, multiple sclerosis, muscle weakness, obesity, osteoarthritis, osteoporosis and other bone diseases, and rheumatoid arthritis. Insufficient levels of vitamin D also increase risk of death from any cause.

Our bodies make vitamin D when our skin is exposed to sunlight without sunscreen, but few people today get enough sun to meet their vitamin D needs. In most of the United States, the sun is not strong enough during winter months to trigger vitamin D production, and during the rest of the year, the sun poses its own risks. In food, cod liver oil, not a popular item today, is the richest source of the nutrient. Although milk and other foods are fortified with vitamin D, the amounts are relatively small. Researchers have estimated that only 4 percent of Americans over age 50 consume enough vitamin D in their diets.

VITAMIN E

Various studies have shown that vitamin E may have a protective effect against hot flashes, PMS and many other conditions, including heart disease, cancer, diabetes, sun damage, brain disorders, eye disorders, pancreatitis (inflammation of the pancreas), frostbite, damage from air pollution, excessive weight loss due to HIV or AIDS, premature aging, anemia and scarring. Although we think of vitamin E as a single nutrient, in food, it's actually a combination of various forms of the vitamin, collectively referred to as tocopherols. For optimum benefits, look for vitamin E and mixed tocopherols, which may be listed together or, vitamin E may be toward the top of the list with mixed tocopherols listed separately, further down.

CALCIUM

In addition to being a key component of healthy bones, calcium is required for breaking up fats, normal transmission of signals through the nervous system, transport of nutrients across cell membranes, muscle contraction, including normal heart rhythm, optimum blood clotting and normal functioning of enzymes and hormones. To utilize the mineral effectively, our bodies require adequate vitamin D and magnesium, and we're more likely to lack these other two nutrients than calcium. Because calcium is added to many foods, including dairy products, orange juice and some cereals, most people need less from supplements than the daily recommended total (1,000 mg up to age 50 and then 1,200 mg). It's wise to check the calcium content of foods you eat routinely and use supplements to cover the shortfall.

While it's important to get enough calcium, it's also possible to get too much. For men, there is some concern that consuming more than 600 mg of calcium from dairy products may contribute to prostate cancer risk. In both men and women, some very preliminary research suggests that taking too much calcium may lead to deposits of the mineral in the arteries. And, too much calcium can cause constipation. Excess sodium, phosphates (found in soda), excess alcohol and smoking cause more calcium to be excreted.

MAGNESIUM

Researchers have estimated that at least half of Americans don't get enough magnesium from their diets, which is not surprising, given that plant foods are the chief food source. Magnesium keeps bones from becoming brittle and is important for the function of muscles, kidneys, the heart and all other organs. It helps to regulate levels of calcium, vitamin D and other essential nutrients and tends to have a relaxing effect, which helps to alleviate muscle cramps and PMS symptoms and to improve sleep. Vitamin B6 is necessary to utilize magnesium efficiently, so it's a good idea to get at least some of the mineral in a multi.

Symptoms of insufficient magnesium may include chocolate cravings, PMS, constipation, depression, low energy levels, learning disabilities, excessive sensitivity to noise or pain, poor appetite or anorexia, headaches, agitation, anxiety, irritability, nausea, vomiting, abnormal heart rhythms, confusion, muscle spasms or cramps, restless leg syndrome, muscle weakness, hyperventilation, insomnia and poor nail growth. The mineral enables the heart and blood vessels to relax and pump blood optimally, and inadequate amounts contribute to high blood pressure and heart disease. Risks for diabetes, osteoporosis and possibly cancer also increase without enough magnesium. Stress can lead to a shortfall because it causes the mineral to be excreted. If you take more than your body can use, magnesium will have a laxative effect, which is easy to remedy by taking a little less.

CHROMIUM

Since the 1950s, chromium has been recognized for its beneficial effect on blood-sugar levels, and indirectly it may help to control weight. Chromium appears to increase sensitivity of cells to insulin, meaning it improves the ability of cells to take in blood sugar and use it as fuel for generating energy. Given that muscle cells' refusal to accept blood sugar is a trigger of hormonal disruption as well as a key contributor to weight gain, chromium plays a key role in helping to restore and maintain balance among hormones. By stabilizing blood sugar, it may also alleviate cravings for sugary and starchy foods and help curb an overzealous appetite. For anyone who is diabetic, dosages of insulin or other medication may need to be adjusted when chromium is taken.

SELENIUM

A trace mineral (meaning it occurs in small quantities), selenium acts as an antioxidant and is required for proper thyroid function and overall wellness. Low levels are associated with higher risk for thyroid malfunction, cancer, heart disease, infection, asthma, infertility among men and women, miscarriage, depression and rheumatoid arthritis. Getting adequate selenium may help to resolve acne and other skin conditions. It works synergistically with vitamin E, so it's a good idea to get your selenium in a multi.

ZINC

Another trace mineral, zinc is found in every cell and required by more than 300 enzymes in the human body for optimum function. It helps insulin do its job, which is critical to keep hormones balanced, and is also an antioxidant. Zinc is necessary for healthy immune function, skin, eyes, fertility, wound healing and overall health. Although our diets tend to be deficient in zinc, too much can create a deficiency of copper and can be toxic. Multis contain copper along with zinc to maintain a balance between the two nutrients. For colds, zinc lozenges can shorten duration and severity of symptoms, and topical zinc products can help to heal cold sores.

IODINE

Also a trace mineral, iodine is necessary for proper thyroid function, and a deficiency may contribute to the formation of fibrocystic breast tissue. Ordinary table salt is enriched with iodine and is the chief source of the nutrient for most

Americans, who typically get approximately 160 to 600 mcg daily from their salt. High-quality multis usually include iodine.

ADDITIONAL BASIC NUTRIENTS

There's only so much that will fit in a multi pill, so fish oil and CoQ10 have to be taken separately. Both are part of the nutritional foundation for overall health and well-being. For anyone who feels strongly about eating only plant-based foods, flaxseed oil can be an alternative to fish oil, although the nutritional composition of the two oils is not identical. One can't assume that benefits of flaxseed oil will equal those of fish oil, as there is not enough evidence to support the premise.

FISH OIL

The omega-3 fatty acids in fish oil cool off inflammation, protect the heart, reduce physical and mental pain, decrease risk for other diseases and premature aging and mitigate uncomfortable symptoms that often appear as hormone levels fluctuate during the course of life. Studies have found that fish oil provides relief from PMS and menstrual pain and reduces the number of hot flashes, feelings of distress, depression and mood swings among women approaching or going through menopause. It may also help with weight loss.

Fish oil plays a key role in preventing or reversing hormonal imbalance triggered by spikes and crashes in blood sugar. The fatty acids in the oil are building blocks of cell membranes, which house receptors, or "doors" that enable cells to receive signals and nutrients, including taking in blood glucose when it is delivered by the hormone insulin. Without healthy cell membranes, cells aren't able to function properly. In contrast to the therapeutic effect of fish oil, unhealthy fats that are prevalent in the typical Western diet can damage cell membranes, cause inflammation and disrupt signals necessary for maintaining hormonal balance and overall health.

Fish oil is our richest source of two specific omega-3 fatty acids: EPA (eicosapentaenoic acid) and DHA (docosahexaenoic acid). Although both nutrients are equally vital for good health, EPA is viewed as the key anti-inflammatory component, and DHA is vital for healthy brain function at all ages and for development of a healthy fetus and child. EPA and DHA are classified as essential nutrients because our bodies don't make them, so diet is our only source.

Studies have found a long list of other fish oil benefits, including: relief from chronic pain; reduced risk of diabetes; mood improvement, including relief from depression, bipolar disorder, schizophrenia and attention deficit disorder among people of all ages; reduction of overly aggressive behavior; a significant decrease in behavioral problems among teens convicted of crimes; healthier skin; relief from inflammatory skin conditions; decreased sun sensitivity and protection against sun burn. Fish oil can also help to prevent or alleviate arthritis, osteoporosis, eating disorders, burns, inflammatory bowel disease, asthma and macular degeneration. On a beauty note, dermatologist Nicholas Perricone, M.D., views fish oil as the closest thing to a facelift in a pill, because the omega-3 fatty acids keep skin hydrated and supple and counteract inflammation that speeds up the aging process.

When looking at different fish oil supplements, be aware that

EPA and DHA, the key omega-3 fatty acids, make up approximately one-third of the oil as it is found in fish. Some products are formulated to have a higher proportion of these fatty acids. Based on the research, the daily amount of a combination of EPA and DHA should be 1,000 mg (1 g). To get that amount from most supplements, you would need to take 3,000 mg (3 g) of fish oil. All reputable manufacturers purify the oil so that it doesn't contain toxins, such as mercury, which may have been present in the fish. To reap the benefits, fish oil needs to be taken on a regular basis.

COQ10 (COENZYME Q10)

Pronounced "co-cue-ten," CoQ10 is found in every cell and is essential for the production of energy that keeps human beings alive. It is used as fuel by the mitochondria, the energy-generating components of cells. Levels of CoQ10 start declining around age 35, paralleling the aging process and contributing to the development of heart disease and other debilitating conditions, including cancer.

As well as being an antioxidant, CoQ10 is used in cell growth and protects against cellular damage that can lead to cancer. Some studies have found a link between low levels of CoQ10 and cancers of the breast, prostate, lung, colon, kidney, head and neck. In combination with other antioxidants and cancer treatments, CoQ10 has helped to shrink cancerous breast tumors. Since breast cancer risk increases significantly after menopause, it makes sense for women to take this supplement.

Among women and men, numerous studies have found that CoQ10 significantly improves health for anyone suffering from heart disease, including congestive heart failure, angina and cardiomyopathy (a diseased heart muscle), and aids in recovery from a heart attack. More than 1,000 heart patients have been participants in these trials. Other research has shown that CoQ10 can help to reduce blood pressure, improve blood-sugar control among diabetics, help to heal gum disease and improve capacity to exercise. Statin drugs, used to lower cholesterol, deplete CoQ10.

Cardiologists report that CoQ10 helps patients in their 80s and 90s maintain a healthy heart and an active life. At a minimum, low CoQ10 levels make it difficult for the human body to produce enough energy for the heart, other organs and muscles to function well. Supplements are the practical way to replenish levels of the nutrient, since organ meats, which very few people eat, are the only significant food source. CoQ10 supplements have been used around the world for more than 20 years and have been found to be safe and beneficial.

FLAXSEED OIL

If you object to consuming any animal-sourced foods or supplements, flaxseed oil is a rich plant source of omega-3 fatty acids. You can't assume that it will provide identical benefits to fish oil, but it's a possible alternative if you believe in eating only foods from the plant kingdom. Flaxseed oil doesn't contain EPA and DHA, the key therapeutic ingredients in fish oil, but it contains a precursor to these, an omega-3 fatty acid called alpha-linolenic acid. The human body has to convert the alpha-linolenic acid in flax to EPA and DHA, and so far, the efficiency of the conversion process is not completely understood. To reap health benefits, get 1 to 2 tablespoons of flaxseed oil daily. It should not be exposed to heat but can be added to salad dressings, smoothies or other foods, or taken as a supplement in capsules. The oil is also a good food source of omega-3 fats for anyone.

TIMING

As a rule, supplements will be utilized more effectively if taken with food, and any ingredients that help your body to generate energy should be taken early in the day. Here are some simple guidelines.

- If your multi consists of one pill, take it with breakfast, and if a daily serving is more than one pill, take half with breakfast and the rest with lunch. It's best not to take multis later in the day as B vitamins improve energy, and there's a chance that they may keep you up if taken late in the day.
- Take CoQ10 in the morning, since it enhances energy production. To absorb it well, take CoQ10 with some food that contains a little fat.
- Take extra vitamin D with your multi so that you don't forget to take it.
- If your daily serving of fish oil consists of several capsules, split these between breakfast, lunch and dinner. Some people find that taking too much fish oil at once makes them burp.
- Extra vitamin C and calcium won't interfere with sleep and can be taken any time, preferably with food.
- For better sleep, take 400 mg of magnesium glycinate or 600 mg of magnesium oxide in the evening.

SHOPPING GUIDE

MULTI

These are some key ingredients to look for in a good quality product. The amounts of each nutrient are a rough guide.

NUTRIENT	APPROXIMATE QUANTITY PER SERVING SIZE
Vitamin A, beta-carotene and other carotenoids	5,000 IU or less of vitamin A; up to 15,000 IU of mixed carotenoids
B vitamins	50 to 100 mg of B1 (thiamine), B2 (riboflavin), B3 (niacin or niacinamide), B5 (pantothenic acid) and B6 (pyridoxine) Up to 1,000 mcg of B12 (cobalamin)
Folic acid	800 mcg
Vitamin C	1,000 to 2,000 mg daily, divided into several doses Up to 5,000 mg during times of stress, from a multi and additional vitamin C supplements
Vitamin D	A total of 1,000 to 2,000 IU daily of the D3 form (cholecalciferol), from a multi and additional vitamin D supplements
Vitamin E	200 to 400 IU of a combination of vitamin E and mixed tocopherols
Calcium	500 mg
Magnesium	at least 250 mg
Chromium	at least 200 mcg
Selenium	200 mcg
Zinc	20 to 40 mg
Iodine	150 to 200 mcg

IN ADDITION TO A MULTI

Some products provide daily servings of a variety of vitamins, minerals and fish oil in a packet-a-day format, rather than a bottle of pills, and the packets may contain everything you need. Otherwise, you will need to add some individual nutrients. For information about antioxidant formulas, see the next page.

Extra vitamin C	Add to your multi daily if needed and take extra C in times of stress.
Extra Vitamin D	Multis don't usually contain adequate amounts so add enough to get 1,000 to 2,000 IU total daily.
Extra Calcium	Aim for 1,000 mg daily up to age 50 and 1,200 mg after that, from a combination of food and supplements. Supplements should only make up for any shortfall from food and you may not need more than the amount in a multi.
Extra Magnesium	Aim to get 400 mg twice daily of the glycinate form or 600 mg twice daily of the oxide form, from a combination of a multi and additional magnesium supplements. If diarrhea occurs, reduce the amount.
Fish Oil	3,000 mg (3 g) and 5,000 mg (5 g) when PMS symptoms begin.
CoQ10	After age 35, take 50 mg or, if you are overweight or have high blood pressure, fatigue, diabetes, any form of heart disease or other illness, take 100 to 200 mg.
Flaxseed Oil (optional)	1 to 2 tablespoons daily or the equivalent in capsule form.

WHAT ABBREVIATIONS REPRESENT:
g: gram (1,000 milligrams)   mcg: microgram
mg: milligram (1,000 micrograms)   IU: International Units

SPECIAL ANTIOXIDANT FORMULAS

Combinations of antioxidants are available from many companies and formulas vary, understandably, since nature produces an enormous variety of antioxidant compounds. The ingredients described in the *Special Antioxidant Formulas* section earlier in this chapter–grape seed extract, Pycnogenol, citrus bioflavonoids and quercetin–work together synergistically but may be difficult to find in one supplement. There are a variety of products with two or three of these ingredients but as the book went to press, we could find only one–Isotonix OPC-3–with all four, and its ingredient list merits some explanation. The label of Isotonix OPC-3 doesn't list quercetin because the product contains red wine extract, and the quercetin is found within the red wine, along with other beneficial antioxidants.

Isotonix OPC-3 is produced by Market America, a company that sells through independent distributors, and is available on many web sites. Be aware that Isotonix is the name of a whole line of supplements, including a number of different antioxidant formulas, but the OPC-3 product is the one that contains the four key antioxidants. To locate it, you can use any search engine or visit www.marketamerica.com and search the site for "OPC-3."

10

SUPPLEMENTS FOR INDIVIDUAL SITUATIONS

Beyond the basics of optimum nutrition, dietary supplements can provide relief in specific situations. These are some of the common conditions for which natural remedies are available.

HOT FLASHES, MOOD SWINGS AND PMS

BLACK COHOSH

With a long history of use for relief from menstrual cramps and menopause symptoms, black cohosh is arguably the most popular herbal remedy for hormonal imbalance. Native Americans originally discovered the benefits of the herb, and today German doctors prescribe black cohosh for menstrual and menopausal difficulties. In the United States, it's available in stores that sell herbal remedies, by itself in pills and tinctures and in women's formulas designed to relieve discomfort associated with the menopausal transition.

Hot flashes, mood swings, night sweats, sleep problems and irritability are among the symptoms for which black cohosh is used. Above and beyond tradition, studies have found that the herb is both effective and safe. For example, one study of 304 women found that black cohosh benefits were similar to those of conventional hormone replacement therapy, especially when the herb was taken soon after symptoms began. Another study, with 64 women, compared the benefits of the herb with those of an estrogen patch. During a three-month period, improvements in hot flashes, anxiety and depression were comparable for both types of treatment. Other research found that for menopausal women, the herb is often helpful in reducing vaginal dryness and thinning of vaginal walls.

Black cohosh does not raise levels of estrogen or other hormones in the body, and it does not increase risk of hormone-related cancers, according to a review of research, which analyzed clinical trials involving a total of approximately 2,800 women. The same review concluded that the herb is a safe and effective alternative to conventional hormone replacement therapy.

Other research has identified several mechanisms that help to explain how black cohosh is different from conventional hormone replacement therapy and why it relieves symptoms of hormonal imbalance.

- It influences the brain's temperature control mechanisms.
- It affects serotonin receptors that influence body temperature.
- It may act on the brain's opiate receptors, which affect hormonal balance and regulate pain, temperature and appetite.

Black cohosh is usually taken for up to six months at a time because there have not been any studies to examine its impact for longer periods. There are no known interactions between the herb and medications. Is it a panacea? No, because individual circumstances vary, and there is no single magic bullet for all women. If you decide to try black cohosh and don't experience improvement within one to two months, discuss other options with your physician. Underlying conditions, such as diabetes, could be triggering or intensifying hot flashes, or medications such as antidepressants could be contributing to symptoms that appear to stem from menopause. Therapeutic amounts vary, depending on the particular formulation of the herb.

GLA (GAMMA-LINOLENIC ACID)

Some women find that GLA, an essential fat, helps to reduce PMS and menopausal symptoms. GLA is a beneficial omega-6 fat, a different type of healthy fat than the omega-3 fats found in fish. The subject can be a bit confusing because processed foods contain omega-6 fats which are unhealthy and promote inflammation. In other words, some omega-6 fats have a negative effect, while others have a positive one, and GLA falls in the positive category. It reduces inflammation and may help to improve eczema, dry eye, osteoporosis (in combination with omega-3 fats), ADHD, rheumatoid arthritis and allergies. GLA may also improve a complication of diabetes, diabetic neuropathy, which causes pain, tingling and numbness in the extremities. GLA is found in evening primrose oil, borage oil and black currant seed oil and is available as an oil or in capsules.

STRESS, MOOD AND SLEEP DIFFICULTIES

HERBAL STRESS BUFFERS

According to the World Health Organization, 80 percent of the world's population currently uses herbs as medicines. Also called botanical medicine, the practice of healing with herbs is older than recorded history. More recently, scientists have started to isolate active ingredients in medicinal plants and test their efficacy. Many clinical trials have shown specific benefits, but because any single herb contains a combination of ingredients, a Western-style method of analyzing the plants has yet to fully reveal the exact way in which they heal. Herbs are often combined, according to time-tested formulas, to provide a specific benefit. One formula that works well for people who feel stressed and wired is Serenagen, a combination of Chinese herbs from Metagenics. It's best used as part of an overall hormone balancing program.

5-HTP

An amino acid, 5-HTP (5-Hydroxytryptophan) naturally raises levels of serotonin, a substance that brain and nerve cells use to communicate. Serotonin is a "feel good" chemical that is naturally present in our bodies, but sometimes in short supply, especially in times of stress. Because of its effect on serotonin, 5-HTP helps to relieve stress, sleep difficulties, anxiety, depression, panic attacks, migraines, tension headaches and stiffness and pain associated with fibromyalgia. It also helps to keep hormones in balance and, for some women, provides some relief from hot flashes. Some studies have also found that 5-HTP spontaneously curbs appetite, especially cravings for carbohydrates or overeating as a result of stress or depression. 5-HTP is available as an individual supplement and in some formulas for stress relief and sleep support. Daily dosages vary from 50 to 100 mg, one to three times daily. It should not be taken with medications that affect serotonin, such as some antidepressants.

L-THEANINE

Another amino acid, l-theanine is believed to be the key ingredient responsible for the relaxing effect of green tea. Studies have found the supplement may improve mood while reducing stress and anxiety and may counteract jitters from too much caffeine. While it promotes relaxation, l-theanine doesn't cause drowsiness and may increase mental alertness, focus and memory. It may be included in formulas designed to improve sleep or counteract stress and is available as an individual supplement.

DIGESTION

DIGESTIVE ENZYMES

Food in its natural state contains enzymes, which we require to break down the food and utilize nutrients, but the enzymes are destroyed by high temperatures in cooking and processing. The result is poor digestion, which can lead to lack of energy, bloating, heartburn, gas, indigestion, constipation, diarrhea and weight gain. Inability to digest can also trigger or contribute to a host of other, seemingly unrelated discomforts, including craving certain foods, thyroid problems, dull or thinning hair, lackluster skin, weak or cracked nails, sleep problems, arthritis or joint pain, depression, mood swings, headaches, ADHD, rashes, hives, hot flashes and PMS.

We need different categories of enzymes to break down different types of foods: protease for digestion of proteins, amylase for carbohydrates and lipase for fats. In addition, there are many other enzymes with more specific roles, such as cellulase for digestion of cellulose, a component of plant fibers found in fruits, vegetables, nuts and grains; invertase for sugar; glucoamylase for maltose, the sugar in grains; and lactase for lactose in dairy products.

If you decide to try digestive enzymes, choose a product from a reputable company with a broad range of enzymes. On the Supplement Facts section of the label, after the name of each enzyme, you'll notice a number and an alphabet soup of letters. The numbers relate to the quantity of food a given enzyme can break down under laboratory conditions, and the letters are acronyms for the exact type of test used to determine the potency of each enzyme. In other words, these details are chemistry speak. If you like, you can use the numbers to compare products. Enzymes should be taken just before meals, according to individual product directions or as recommended by your physician.

WEIGHT-LOSS SUPPORT

L-CARNITINE

Unlike weight-loss supplements that promise a quick fix, l-carnitine is a nutrient we use all the time to sustain energy production, a process that must work efficiently for a healthy weight to be achieved and maintained. It's especially important for energy production in the heart and muscles and works synergistically with CoQ10, one of the basic supplements covered in the previous chapter.

Found chiefly in red meat, l-carnitine gets its name from "carnus," the Latin word for flesh. It's used by our bodies to turn fat from our food into energy, delivering fatty acids to cells and removing toxic waste, which is a byproduct of the energy-generating process. Studies have found that l-carnitine improves the function of the heart, arteries, nervous system and brain and enhances the ability to perform exercise. It may also help to relieve anorexia, chronic fatigue, diphtheria, hypoglycemia, male infertility, muscular dystrophy and Rett syndrome, a neurological disorder. Research also shows it may aid in recovery from heart disease and help to reduce complications of diabetes by protecting nerve endings from damage due to the disease. Symptoms of l-carnitine deficiency may include fatigue, weakness, chest or muscle pain, low blood pressure and confusion. A daily amount of 500 mg can support a healthy diet and exercise.

VAGINAL YEAST INFECTIONS

PROBIOTICS

Found in yogurt, keefir and dietary supplements, probiotics are "friendly" bacteria that protect women against vaginal yeast infections by restoring an optimum balance among organisms naturally present in the vagina. The same bacteria also keep the intestinal tract healthy, improving digestion and helping to reduce inflammation and improve immune function. When choosing yogurt, look for products with a variety of live cultures (only live cultures contain beneficial bacteria) but without added sugar or artificial flavorings. It's best to buy unflavored yogurt and add fresh or frozen fruit, or eat it plain. Or, take probiotic supplements. Individual needs for probiotics vary.

CONSTIPATION

FLAXSEED

For thousands of years, flaxseed has been used to relieve constipation; more recently, research has shown that, compared to psyllium seed, ground flaxseed produces less bloating and abdominal pain. Because of its high fiber content, flaxseed can also help prevent heart disease and may help control levels of cholesterol and blood sugar. For relief from constipation, take 1 tablespoon of ground flaxseed two to three times daily, with plenty of water.

URINARY TRACT INFECTIONS

CRANBERRY

By inhibiting the ability of harmful bacteria to adhere to the walls of the bladder, cranberry enables those bacteria to be washed away, thereby helping to prevent or relieve urinary tract infections. Research has also found that cranberry reduces harmful bacteria in the urine and can help to reduce chronic bladder infections among postmenopausal women. In studies, both supplements and juice have produced results if taken in sufficient quantities.

To get the benefits, you need to drink 8 to 16 ounces of pure cranberry juice daily or take 300 to 400 mg of an extract twice per day. If you decide on cranberry juice, choose one without sweeteners or other additives and add a little agave syrup or pure apple juice for natural sweetness. Sweetening with stevia, a very sweet herb with no calories, is another option. Or mix the cranberry juice in a smoothie with fresh apple.

PREVENTION OF HORMONE-RELATED CANCERS

INDOLE-3-CARBINOL

Frequently abbreviated as I3C, Indole-3-Carbinol is a substance derived from cruciferous vegetables such as broccoli, cabbage and cauliflower, foods known to protect against cancer. I3C is a valuable supplement for prevention of breast, cervical and other hormone-related cancers, especially if a pap smear reveals abnormal growth of cells (dysplasia), or if you have fibroids, breast cysts or heavy bleeding.

I3C alters the metabolism of estrogen, converting it from a form that is associated with breast, cervical, endometrial and prostate cancers to a weaker form that doesn't increase cancer risk. Research also shows it may reduce the odds of breast cancer triggered by environmental toxins that have an estrogenic effect (for common sources of toxins see chapter 7). In lab studies, I3C has also demonstrated an ability to inhibit growth of human papilloma virus, cysts and precancerous lesions, to stop growth of cancer cells and to cause cancerous cells to self-destruct. In human trials, the amount of I3C taken was most often 200 to 400 mg daily.

PAIN

Pain medications mask pain. In contrast, dietary supplements are designed to be used as a foundation for optimum nutrition and to address specific situations underlying various types of physical pain and other symptoms. In the supplements covered above, relief from pain is one possible benefit of black cohosh, gamma-linolenic acid, 5-HTP, digestive enzymes and l-carnitine.

However, if you are in pain, that doesn't mean you should you rush out, buy and start taking all of these.

In many cases, optimum health requires assessing your overall situation, determining what may be triggering pain or other symptoms, and addressing those causes. For example, inflammation, a basic contributing factor to various types of pain, develops due to a combination of factors, including excess weight, a pro-inflammatory diet, lack of physical activity and stress. Knee pain due to osteoarthritis, a common reason for pain medication, is often relieved by weight loss. Even slight weight gain places a much greater burden on the knees, raising the risk for osteoarthritis, hastening progression of the disease and increasing the potential need for eventual knee replacement. According to the Arthritis Foundation, for every pound you gain, the knees receive three pounds of added stress. In contrast, research shows that when an overweight person loses 11 pounds, the risk for osteoarthritis is cut in half.

Depending on your personal circumstances, it's quite possible that one or more of the above remedies, in combination with a sound eating plan, basic supplements, the right exercise and stress management may resolve your situation quite quickly. If that doesn't happen, you can work with a physician who specializes in helping patients to achieve optimum wellness.

11

BIOIDENTICAL HORMONES

Mention bioidentical hormones, and many people will respond with a blank stare. What kind of hormones? Bioidentical ones, which are designed to be utilized by our bodies just like the hormones we produce internally and can improve our overall state of well-being and quality of life.

When employed correctly under the care of a qualified physician, such hormones relieve hot flashes, other symptoms of menopause and a variety of manifestations of broader hormonal imbalance that can occur long before "the change." And they produce these benefits without harmful side effects.

Bioidentical hormones are quite different from those used in traditional hormone replacement therapy, or HRT, which has been found to increase risk for breast cancer and heart disease. However, because the difference between HRT and bioidentical hormones is not well understood, the mere mention of any kind of hormone therapy can put people on guard. Consider this chapter a basic primer that aims to clarify some of the most common sources of misunderstanding on the subject.

If you're not familiar with bioidentical hormones, don't feel as though you're "out of the loop." Most physicians are in the same boat. While this type of hormone therapy has been used for many years, it isn't part of the usual treatment in today's health-care system, which focuses on treatment and early detection of disease. Bioidentical hormones are part of a new frontier of medicine that has a broader goal: helping us achieve and maintain an optimum state of well-being for as long as we live.

Be aware that there is some controversy associated with this subject for several reasons: media reports frequently omit or misrepresent scientific evidence supporting the safety of bioidentical hormone therapy; financial interests in the pharmaceutical and health-care industries influence dissemination of information to physicians; medical schools don't train physicians to provide care that will restore and maintain patients' well-being; and today's health-care system revolves around cookie-cutter, one-size-fits-all medicating of symptoms rather than treating the whole person.

Where does this leave you? Quite possibly, confused and frustrated. Countless women have gone to their doctors with symptoms that were ruining their lives, only to be told, "Your tests are normal." By conventional medical standards, their tests really were "normal," because the tests and doctors' examinations were designed to detect disease, and nothing short of disease. In essence, those women were told, "Go home, and don't come back until you have something that can be conveniently labeled and medicated, or surgically removed."

Again, where does this leave you? Quite simply, you have the responsibility to take care of yourself in your day-to-day life and to search for and seek out whatever care you require. And you need to be armed with knowledge. When making your own choices, it's helpful to have an overview of what science has dis-

MANIFESTATIONS OF HORMONAL DECLINE	BENEFITS OF BIOIDENTICAL HORMONE THERAPY
Hot flashes	Relief from hot flashes
Sleep disturbances	Improved sleep
Decreased energy	Improved energy
Depressed or unstable mood	Improved mood
Loss of sex drive	Improved libido
Increased fat	Weight loss
Decreased muscle	Improved body composition
Thinner skin	Improved skin
Decreased memory and mental function	Improved mental function Reduced risk of osteoporosis, Alzheimer's and heart disease

covered about hormone therapy and to know that some physicians are trained to find out what is wrong when conventional tests are "normal" but the patient needs help.

TERMINOLOGY

The meanings of words and phrases relating to hormone use are somewhat muddled. To avoid perpetuating confusion, here's an explanation of some key terms you will see in this chapter.

BIOIDENTICAL HORMONES

Because bioidentical is a term coined fairly recently, physicians who are unfamiliar with it may, in defense of their own ignorance, sometimes express skepticism about the validity of the word. New terminology is part of the rapid evolution of today's culture, and keeping up with new concepts and terms can be challenging. Just a few years ago, how many people would have understood this conversation: "Is that restaurant any good?" "I don't know; I'll Google it."

Bioidentical is a combination of "bio," which means life, and "identical." It literally means "identical to life." In pronunciation, it's almost like two words: "bio (as in "Do you have a bio?") identical." When a hormone is bioidentical, it is built, or structured, just like a hormone produced within a human body. Consequently, when we ingest such a hormone, it is accepted as though it came from one of our own glands.

To recap an analogy from chapter 1: The concept of a jigsaw puzzle helps to illustrate the difference between hormones that are bioidentical and those that are not. In a normal puzzle, the pieces will fit if you put them in the right places. That's how bioidentical hormones work in our bodies: they fit. Hormones that are not bioidentical are like misshapen jigsaw pieces. When they come out of the box, they look like legitimate parts of the puzzle, but when you find the spot where each one should belong, these misfits are not an exact match. They have extra parts jutting out, and these overlap somewhat with adjoining pieces. The spaces are covered, but the whole puzzle won't lie flat, and the picture is distorted.

In a physical sense, hormones that are not bioidentical act like misshapen jigsaw pieces inside the human body, resulting in more risks than benefits. With bioidentical hormones, the jigsaw pieces fit, producing benefits rather than risks.

"SYNTHETIC" HORMONES

Many hormone preparations are not bioidentical, meaning they are not structurally identical to those produced by our bodies. As an example, some estrogen prescriptions are formulated from the estrogen in pregnant mares' urine. If a vet was treating a female horse, that hormone would be bioidentical for the animal, but it is different from the estrogen produced by a human body. In other prescriptions, hormones are chemically formulated to be structurally different from our own. And, some prescriptions that are not bioidentical are made from plants. Sometimes, "synthetic" is used to describe all hormone products that are not bioidentical, and this leads to confusion because we don't think of plants as being synthetic.

Structure, rather than source materials, is what distinguishes bioidentical hormones, because structure determines whether or not a particular hormone formulation is a "perfect match" for our bodies. While plants are found in nature, the structure of some hormone products manufactured from plant materials is not bioidentical. However, all bioidentical hormones are made from plants.

HRT

This is the common abbreviation for hormone replacement therapy. In research performed in the United States, HRT has traditionally referred to treatment with hormones that are not bioidentical, and in this chapter, it is used in the same way. More specifically, when mentioned below, HRT is referring to a combination of estrogen and progesterone hormone replacement prescriptions that are not bioidentical.

BHRT

An abbreviation for "bioidentical hormone replacement therapy," BHRT is another relatively new term. As it implies, it means treatment with bioidentical hormones. If HRT and BHRT seem like confusing pots of alphabet soup, you could think of the "B" in BHRT as an acronym for "better." Research described later in this chapter shows that BHRT does not pose health risks and conveys more health benefits than HRT.

HRT HEALTH RISKS AND PANIC

Until May 31, 2002, the medical community viewed HRT both as a treatment for hot flashes and as a prescription to reduce risk for heart disease among postmenopausal women. Then, on that fateful spring day, experts who routinely review the safety of clinical trials reached some surprising conclusions. In a study of more than 16,000 women, which was part of a larger research project called the Women's Health Initiative, HRT significantly increased health risks. Compared to women taking a placebo, those using HRT (estrogen and progesterone, in hormone prescriptions that were not bioidentical) experienced the following:

- 41 percent increase in strokes
- 29 percent increase in heart attacks
- A doubling of the rates of blood clots
- 22 percent increase in total cardiovascular disease
- 26 percent increase in breast cancer

The study also found that HRT produced some benefits:

- 37 percent reduction in cases of colorectal cancer
- One-third reduction in hip fracture rates
- 24 percent reduction in total fractures

Despite some benefits, safety experts concluded that the risks of HRT were too great, and the trial was immediately stopped to avoid further harm. In July 2002, the *Journal of the American Medical Association* posted the research results on its web site, a week before publication in the print journal, due to the importance of these findings. This journal rarely takes such action. Ever since, HRT has been a confusing and controversial topic.

Further evaluation of data from the same trial showed that health risks were greatest among women who began HRT years after menopause, and risks were somewhat lower among those who began treatment when menopausal symptoms first appeared. Other studies have found that ingesting hormones through the skin, using creams or patches, does not pose the same degree of risk as hormones in pill form, even when such prescriptions are not bioidentical. However, millions of women discarded their HRT prescriptions in 2002 and never filled them again.

In the years that followed, rates of breast cancer among postmenopausal women declined substantially, but the reasons for this positive development were disputed. Although the trend correlated with many women ceasing HRT after the startling research results, some experts posed the theory that, perhaps, fewer women were getting mammograms and therefore less

> ## PROGESTERONE VS. PROGESTINS
>
> These two terms may look or sound similar but they describe hormone preparations which are distinctly different in terms of structure, function, benefits and risks. Progesterone is a hormone our bodies produce and may be used as a bioidentical hormone, also called progesterone, to remedy hormonal imbalance. In contrast, progestins are a family of hormones which are not bioidentical. In clinical trials, progestins have uniformly been found to increase risk for breast cancer. However, research has shown that bioidentical progesterone either does not affect risk for breast cancer or decreases risk. Sometimes, these two terms are erroneously used interchangeably, particularly in news stories.

breast cancer was being detected. However, later research disproved this theory.

Since the 2002 HRT study, analysis of other data from the Women's Health Initiative, published in the *New England Journal of Medicine* in February 2009, concluded that declining rates of breast cancer were predominantly related to a decrease in the use of HRT. The same study also found that in longer-term use of HRT, after the fifth year, risk of breast cancer doubles each year that such prescriptions (which are not bioidentical) continue to be used.

BIOIDENTICAL HORMONE RESEARCH

Treatment with bioidentical hormones has a different impact on health risks and well-being, when compared with HRT. Take a look at some research results.

- A study of more than 54,000 postmenopausal women in France compared risk of breast cancer among women using HRT or bioidentical hormones for nearly three years. Risk for breast cancer increased by up to 70 percent among women taking progestins, forms of progesterone that are not bioidentical. Among those taking bioidentical progesterone, risk decreased by 10 percent.
- A longer-term French study tracked more than 80,000 postmenopausal women for just over eight years, comparing breast-cancer risk among women using estrogen and bioidentical progesterone or progestins. Risk increased by up to 90 percent among those using progestins (which are not bioidentical) but did not increase among women using bioidentical progesterone.
- At the Mayo Clinic, a study of 176 women compared quality of life associated with use of bioidentical progesterone or progestins. Researchers found that when using bioidentical progesterone, women experienced significantly more improvement in a number of areas, including hot flashes, sleep, sex, depression, anxiety and menstrual patterns.
- In Texas, a study of 150 women between the ages of 30 and 70 examined the impact of different types of hormone therapy on risk for heart disease. The women, who were either postmenopausal or were experiencing symptoms associated with menopause, received one of two treatments: bioidentical hormones customized for

their own personal needs, based on lab tests, or HRT (which is not bioidentical) and additional medications to control health risks and symptoms such as pain, depression and elevated blood sugar. The latter type of treatment is typical in medicine today. After 12 months, the women receiving bioidentical hormones had uniformly lowered their risk for heart disease, with healthier levels of blood pressure, blood sugar and triglycerides (a blood fat measured when cholesterol levels are tested), and experienced greater relief from depression, anxiety and pain. Unlike HRT, the bioidentical hormone treatment did not increase blood clots or inflammation.

- A review of nearly 200 studies concluded that, compared to treatment with HRT, bioidentical hormones were more effective in relieving menopausal symptoms and reduced risk for breast cancer and heart disease.

We all like our clothes, undergarments and rings to fit. That's what bioidentical hormones do: they fit. In more technical terms, hormones deliver messages to cellular receptors, which are like tiny little doors on cells. Bioidentical hormones fit perfectly through the doors, but those that are not bioidentical are like oddly shaped, alien creatures that get stuck, and then manage to squeeze through but not without causing some peripheral damage.

THE BASIC STEPS OF BHRT

Typical Western medicine aims to treat symptoms with medication. For example, if a woman tells her doctor that she's experiencing hot flashes, mood swings and sleep problems, minutes later, she will most likely leave the office with prescriptions for HRT plus an antidepressant and a sleep medication. This is quite different from the goal of BHRT, which is to bring about a state of well-being by restoring balance among hormones.

BHRT is a treatment performed by medical doctors with specialized training in the subject. It begins with lab tests to measure levels of several hormones, which usually include estrogen, progesterone, testosterone, cortisol and thyroid hormone. In addition, tests usually include fasting blood sugar and may include cholesterol and other traditional health markers, depending on the individual situation. At the same time, the patient provides information about his or her symptoms and state of health (see *Symptom Questionnaire*).

Once all this information is collected, the doctor and patient spend some time together, discussing test results and identifying related lifestyle factors, and the patient receives a program that may include a prescription for one or more bioidentical hormones, nutritional supplements, and guidelines for dietary changes, exercise and stress management. This initial visit usually takes an hour. Yes, a whole hour during which a doctor and patient actually communicate about the patient's situation and how to improve it. It's a two-way street, a team effort with the goal of helping the patient to achieve a state of well-being.

As an example of how this may work, the woman above, with hot flashes, mood swings and sleep problems, could have high levels of stress in her life that contribute to an imbalance of estrogen, progesterone, testosterone, cortisol and thyroid hormone, in addition to experiencing a menopausal transition. Does this

SYMPTOM QUESTIONNAIRE

These are the types of questions you will be asked before your first visit with a physician who is qualified to provide bioidentical hormone therapy.

- Are you under a significant amount of stress?
- Do you feel as though you're aging rapidly?
- Are your menstrual cycles regular, irregular or non-existent?
- Have you had a hysterectomy?
- Have one or both of your ovaries been removed?
- Are you pregnant?

Do you have any of these conditions?

- acne
- allergies
- bone loss
- fibrocystic breasts
- fibromyalgia
- goiter
- high blood pressure
- high cholesterol
- high triglycerides
- low blood pressure
- low blood sugar
- uterine fibroids

Are you experiencing any of these symptoms?

- aches and pains
- anxiety
- bleeding changes
- breast tenderness
- constipation
- decreased libido
- decreased muscle size
- decreased stamina
- decreased sweating
- depression
- fatigue in the evening
- fatigue in the morning
- feeling cold for no apparent reason
- feeling tearful
- foggy thinking
- hair becoming dry or brittle
- hair growth increasing on your face or body
- hair loss from the scalp
- headaches

Are you experiencing any of these symptoms?

- hearing loss
- heart palpitations
- hoarseness
- hot flashes
- incontinence
- increased urges to urinate
- infertility problems
- irritability
- memory lapses
- mood swings
- nails breaking easily or becoming brittle
- nervousness

- night sweats
- rapid heartbeat
- sensitivity to chemicals
- sleep disturbances
- slow pulse rate
- sugar cravings
- swollen or puffy eyes or face
- thinning skin
- vaginal dryness
- water retention
- weight gain in the hips
- weight gain in the waist

mean she would automatically get prescriptions for five hormones? No. Nothing would be prescribed "automatically."

Her tests, symptoms, diet, use of dietary supplements, exercise habits and stressful life situations would all be discussed. The doctor would listen and take into account her particular circumstances, immediate concerns and longer-term goals. While relief from hot flashes may be one objective, she may be even more concerned about feeling lethargic or exhausted, or lacking enthusiasm for life, and the hormonal and lifestyle factors underlying these would all have to be addressed, as well as the hot flashes.

Equally important, the doctor would also find out what types of lifestyle changes are—or aren't—realistic. Some people exercise too intensely or for too long, while others don't exercise at all, and a dietary change that could be easy for one person would be extremely difficult for another. The dialogue would be an honest, two-way conversation, with the patient learning new ways to improve her situation. She may walk out with a prescription for one or more bioidentical hormones, and a nutritional supplement and lifestyle program.

Six months later, or earlier if needed, the patient will redo some of her tests and see her doctor again. This time, they may only need a half-hour to review her progress and tests and to determine the next steps. If it sounds as though this doctor's office is on another, gentler planet, rest assured that space travel is not required. You can check the Appendix for where to find a physician who practices medicine this way in your area.

12

FREQUENTLY ASKED QUESTIONS

For most people, the idea of restoring harmony among our hormones is new and unfamiliar territory, and it's easy to focus on hormone therapy. To keep things in context, remember that your hormones are affected by how you live every day, and any type of bioidentical hormone treatment from a qualified physician is designed to work in concert with a healthy lifestyle.

A hormone prescription is easy to use, but it doesn't replace the need for healthy food, adequate nutrients, sensible exercise and stress management. That said, the answers to these frequently asked questions provide some additional information about situations in which bioidentical hormone therapy may be used and how the process works.

WHAT IS ADRENAL FATIGUE?

One of the functions of the adrenal glands is to produce the hormone cortisol. Adrenal fatigue is a depletion of normal cortisol levels due to prolonged stress that eventually surpasses these glands' ability to respond. Symptoms of low cortisol include severe morning fatigue and difficulty getting out of bed in the morning, difficulty concentrating, difficulty making decisions, anxiety, depression, feelings of being overwhelmed and symptoms of low blood sugar, which may include feeling dizzy or weak.

Many people with adrenal fatigue have a long history of stressful events that they had previously been able to "handle" but no longer can. They often note an insidious onset of fatigue and a decreasing ability to handle stress. In such situations, many individuals begin to blame themselves, mistakenly believing that they are just getting lazy, or they become concerned that they are suffering from depression. They don't realize that the culprit may be adrenal fatigue, which is not the same as Addison's disease or adrenal failure.

Treatment for adrenal fatigue requires a great deal of cooperation between a qualified physician and patient; they need to be able to work together as a team. Lifestyle treatments include getting enough sleep (try to be in bed by 10 p.m.), limiting your exposure to computers and television just before bed and decreasing stress in personal relationships, at work or in any other stressful area of life. Dietary treatments include limiting sugars, white flour and caffeine as well as getting adequate lean proteins and complex carbohydrates such as vegetables. It is also important to maintain stable levels of blood sugar by eating a little bit every two to three hours. Nutritional support includes multivitamins, antioxidants, B vitamins, vitamin C and magnesium.

Many physicians and patients also utilize a combination of herbs and glandular products to help support the adrenal glands as they heal. In the most severe cases, where the activities of daily life are affected, bioidentical cortisol could be used in the short term, along with diet, lifestyle and nutritional interventions.

WHY IS THYROID HORMONE TESTED?

Thyroid hormone is very important for our metabolism and

energy levels. Symptoms of thyroid deficiency include fatigue, weight gain, constipation, dry skin, foggy thinking, heavy menstrual periods and fluid retention. By some estimates, up to one in seven adults have some level of thyroid deficiency. The tough part is that many of these deficiencies may be missed because conventional thyroid hormone tests are looking for disease states rather than non-optimum levels of thyroid hormone. In BHRT, the goal is well-being, and testing and treatment are done to achieve that goal. Treatment of low thyroid function involves nutrition, including adequate selenium, vitamin A and iodine, and hormone therapy designed for the individual. For optimum thyroid function, the adrenal glands also have to be functioning properly. Otherwise, treating the thyroid when adrenal function is impaired will make a person feel worse.

ISN'T TESTOSTERONE A DANGEROUS STEROID?

The word "steroid" doesn't mean a performance-enhancing drug. Rather, it describes a family of hormones our bodies make from building blocks found in cholesterol. Estrogen, progesterone and cortisol, as well as testosterone, are steroid hormones.

In "anabolic steroids," which are outlawed from sports, testosterone is used in dangerously high doses to build muscular strength and volume, and this type of hormone use is hazardous. For one thing, it can override the body's ability to produce its own testosterone and other hormones, causing problems for many years after anabolic steroid use is discontinued. The fact that anabolic steroids are usually not bioidentical contributes further to their danger. (Damage caused by anabolic steroids can be remedied with BHRT.)

WHAT SEX HORMONES DO FOR WOMEN

Estrogen
- Performs over 400 functions in the female body
- Maintains memory, mood, and muscles
- Protects against heart disease
- Maintains bone and protects against osteoporosis

Progesterone
- Balances the effects of estrogen
- Protects against heart disease
- Has a calming effect and enhances mood
- Balances blood sugar and thyroid function
- Rebuilds bone

Testosterone
- Builds muscles and promotes muscle tone
- Increases energy and libido
- Enhances sense of well-being
- Strengthens bone

Both men and women naturally produce testosterone and require optimum levels of the hormone to function well. In bioidentical hormone therapy, testosterone, where necessary according to individual test results, is prescribed in small doses to restore balance among hormones, and this type of use improves overall health rather than posing risks.

ARE BIOIDENTICAL HORMONES NATURAL?

Yes, but not in the way most people think. One of the definitions of "natural" in *Webster's Third New International Dictionary* is this: "closely resembling the object imitated: true to life." In hormone therapy, the objects being imitated are the hormones made by our bodies. Since bioidentical hormones are identical in structure to our internally produced hormones, they are natural in this sense. In contrast, hormones that are not bioidentical have a significantly different structure from that of our own hormones and are not natural per the Webster's definition.

Many people think bioidentical hormones are natural because they are made from plants, and this line of reasoning can lead to confusion, because some of the hormone prescriptions that are not bioidentical are also made from plants. In both types of formulations, the plant ingredients are manipulated in a lab, by human beings, to make the end product. To avoid confusion, the word "bioidentical" is used to describe the key characteristic of hormones that are structured in the same way as those produced by our bodies.

HOW QUICKLY DO BIOIDENTICAL HORMONES WORK?

Many people experience some relief from hot flashes and other symptoms within days. It's realistic to expect a noticeable improvement within two to three weeks, with benefits continuing to increase over a longer period of time. In some situations, such as severe hormonal imbalance that began after the birth of a child decades ago, it will take longer for a full restoration of balance.

WHY ARE TESTS NEEDED?

It isn't possible to say that a given symptom always stems from a lack of a specific hormone. For example, sleep problems could result from non-optimum levels of estrogen, progesterone, and cortisol, or some combination of those hormones. In terms of basic functions, progesterone initiates sleep, and estrogen helps sleep to continue uninterrupted. However, cortisol malfunctions can interfere with restful sleep and cause debilitating fatigue first thing in the morning and disturbing fluctuations in energy levels at other times of day. Malfunction in thyroid hormone can also cause fatigue.

Sound confusing? It can be because a symptom can be caused by a combination of hormonal factors, and the wrong treatment can make things worse. That's why lab tests are so important.

HOW ARE TESTS DONE?

Saliva, blood and urine tests may be used, depending on which hormones or other health markers are being measured. For example, cortisol levels are often measured with saliva tests at four different times of the day, as levels of the hormone naturally fluctuate during a 24-hour period, and the pattern provides valuable data. It would be difficult for most people to have blood drawn four times during one day, and the process itself could raise levels of stress and, therefore, increase levels of cortisol and interfere with the accuracy of the tests. A significant body of research has validated saliva testing as an accurate method of measurement when used appropriately. A qualified physician will determine which types of tests are required, based on an individual's personal situation.

DO I NEED A PRESCRIPTION?

Yes. Hormone preparations are not available over the counter, with the exception of some very low-dose progesterone products, which are discussed in detail in *Dr. John Lee's Hormone Balance Made Simple*. However, wild yam preparations, which are sometimes marketed as a natural alternative for progesterone for menopause relief, are not the same substance as progesterone, and cannot be expected to deliver the same benefits. Keep in mind that hormone therapy is not a do-it-yourself affair, and working with a qualified physician and getting the right prescription, for the right amount of the hormone or hormones you need at a given point in your life, is what brings about the best results.

IN WHAT FORM ARE BIOIDENTICAL HORMONES TAKEN?

Where an individual needs one or more of the sex hormones–estrogen, progesterone or testosterone–these are often applied on the skin, as creams or gels. Vaginal creams are also used, when appropriate. Other prescriptions may deliver a hormone in a lozenge or pill, and in some cases, pellets are inserted under the skin to release one or more hormones over a period of several months.

Where thyroid hormone or cortisol are required, these are taken as pills or capsules. For optimum benefits, there is no one-size-fits-all solution. Determining the best type of delivery system for each individual is part of the physician's role in bioidentical hormone therapy.

HOW MUCH DO BIOIDENTICAL HORMONES COST?

The cost depends on your personal needs. Per day, hormone prescription costs can range from 20 cents to nearly $1 per hormone. The exact cost depends upon several factors, including the dose required and the pricing structure of a specific pharmacy. To find pharmacies that specialize in filling bioidentical hormone prescriptions, have strict quality control procedures and work with many health plans, see *Compounding Pharmacies* in the Appendix.

CAN BIOIDENTICAL HORMONE PRESCRIPTIONS BE FILLED AT MY LOCAL PHARMACY?

There are two ways in which bioidentical hormones can be manufactured: customized for an individual, based on a doctor's prescription, or mass produced by a pharmaceutical company. The mass-produced varieties have specific doses and combinations of hormones, and may contain ingredients that some people are allergic to, such as peanut oil. If one of these mass-produced hormones fits your needs, then you can get your prescription filled at a local pharmacy. However, if you need a customized prescription, this can be made by a pharmacy that is specially skilled and equipped to fill such prescriptions. Large chain pharmacies do not make customized prescriptions.

HOW CAN I TELL IF A MASS-PRODUCED HORMONE PRESCRIPTION IS BIOIDENTICAL?

Some mass-produced hormones are bioidentical, while others are not. In some cases, mass-produced prescriptions contain more than one hormone, and one of these may be bioidentical while the other is not, so it can get pretty confusing.

If your doctor is not well versed in the subject, he or she will probably not know which brands are bioidentical and won't consider that it makes any difference. In this case, you will have to do your own research. See *Bioidentical Hormone Brands* in the Appendix for a list of mass-produced brands that are bioidentical. To receive updates as more information becomes available, visit www.hormoneharmony.org.

CAN MY REGULAR DOCTOR PRESCRIBE BIOIDENTICAL HORMONES?

Yes, but in a limited way. For example, if your doctor gives you a prescription to replace estrogen and progesterone, one or both of those prescribed hormone formulations could, possibly, be bioidentical. However, there could be a few glitches: The dose may not be right for you, because most doctors don't test to determine patients' individual needs. And, routine medical care doesn't take into account the other key hormones, such as thyroid, testosterone and cortisol, nor does it address nutrition or other lifestyle issues that affect your overall hormonal picture. Consequently, the estrogen and progesterone may or may not lead you to your best possible state of health.

WHAT IS A COMPOUNDED PRESCRIPTION?

Compounding is the process of combining ingredients to make a customized prescription that is not available in a mass-produced version in a strength or form needed by a patient. In addition to bioidentical hormones, medications are compounded for a variety of other types of treatment. One could call the process "mixing," but pharmaceutical compounding isn't the same thing as making a cake batter in your kitchen, so it deserves a special name.

In compounding, the bioidentical hormone ingredients

used are FDA approved, and pharmacists who compound them require specialized training and equipment. The final product must meet very precise standards of purity and potency, per a doctor's prescription. When individuals require formulations of bioidentical hormones that are not available in mass-produced versions, compounded prescriptions can meet their needs.

ARE COMPOUNDING PHARMACIES REGULATED?

All pharmacies, including those who specialize in compounding prescriptions, are regulated by state licensing boards and must meet set standards. Pharmacists must be licensed and are required to meet specific levels of continuing education, just like doctors and other licensed health-care professionals.

However, not all pharmacists have specialized training in compounding customized prescriptions, and it is vital to work with those who do. To ensure consistently high-quality products, reputable compounding pharmacies insist that their personnel have specialized training in compounding, use state-of-the-art equipment, and abide by well-defined quality assurance standards and procedures, including having random samples of compounded prescriptions frequently tested by an independent lab. This way, compounded prescriptions can meet the highest standards of safety, purity and accurate potency.

In addition, a compounding pharmacy should always work with your doctor, as that is who issues your prescription. The pharmacies listed in *Compounding Pharmacies* in the Appendix meet these criteria and are licensed to fill prescriptions throughout the United States.

IS BHRT COVERED BY HEALTH INSURANCE?

Individual health plans vary considerably, from those that cover very little to those that pay for significant portions of testing and BHRT treatment costs. With the number and diversity of insurance plans, it's impossible to say what yours may cover. The costs break down into these three components:

TESTS: Many health plans will cover at least some of these, based on your condition, other recent claims and policy.

PRESCRIPTIONS: Most health plans that include drug coverage will pay for prescriptions for mass-produced bioidentical hormones, minus your co-pay, as with any prescription. In the case of customized, compounded prescriptions, many plans cover these as well. However, compounded hormones sometimes cost less than a co-pay. A compounding pharmacy that works with a lot of health insurance plans can help to keep your costs as low as possible.

DOCTOR VISITS: Some progressive health plans provide ample benefits but many cover only a small portion of office-visit fees.

As a rule, doctors who have the specialized medical training to provide BHRT will give patients the treatment codes required for presenting a claim for reimbursement to a health plan. However, a physician trained in BHRT spends much more time, one-on-one, with a patient than a conventional physician, and health-care plans are not designed to cover this personalized type of service. Office visits covered by insurance plans usually last no more than a few minutes, and that's all health plans are usually willing to pay for. This situation is a big contributor to the problems in our health-care system.

If optimum health is your goal, this is an example of what you can expect to spend in your first year: approximately $400 for an initial consultation with a qualified physician, $250 for a follow-up consultation six months later, plus tests and prescriptions. However, physicians' costs vary, depending on where you live. Initial tests cost between $400 and $500. Follow-up testing is usually much less and depends on individual needs, as do costs of prescriptions. These are estimates of total costs, so any coverage from a health plan would reduce these amounts.

As mentioned above, hormone prescriptions can range from 20 cents to nearly $1 per hormone, per day. Nutritional supplements are never covered by health plans and costs vary considerably, based on individual needs. All told, the total cost, before any insurance reimbursement or coverage, is likely to range between $1,000 and $2,000 during the first year.

If you're taken aback, keep in mind that many people spend much more than $2,000 annually on car payments or, in some cases, on home entertainment. Unlike our bodies, cars are replaceable, and even the biggest screen, highest definition TV isn't so much fun if you're not in good health. Given the return on your investment, the costs of taking care of yourself are not very high.

DO I HAVE TO TAKE BIOIDENTICAL HORMONES FOR THE REST OF MY LIFE?

There is certainly no requirement to do so. Many women (and

men) today are facing a hormonal crisis that has developed during the previous decades of their lives, and additional, age-related fluctuations in hormone levels are accentuating a longer-term imbalance. This situation needs to be addressed with nutrition, stress management, exercise and, where necessary, bioidentical hormone therapy.

The goal is to restore and perpetuate well-being. If you want to feel good and function well for the rest of your life, there are definitely certain lifestyle requirements. It's virtually impossible to abuse a human body for decades with unhealthy food, inadequate nutrients, chronically high stress levels and little or no physical activity without experiencing adverse consequences.

Bioidentical hormone therapy may be necessary as a temporary measure to restore balance, but how long it is continued always depends upon individual circumstances and choices. By adopting a way of life that fosters optimum functioning of hormones and other systems in your body, as well as your mind and spirit, you can enjoy a long and fulfilling life.

WHERE DO I FIND A QUALIFIED DOCTOR?

As a first step, you can check *How to Find Qualified Physicians* in the Appendix. If that doesn't help you locate a doctor in your area, you can check with the pharmacies that are also listed in the Appendix, as these deal with many physicians who are qualified to provide BHRT throughout the country. When considering a doctor, ask about that individual's training related to hormone therapy and specialties in which he or she is board certified.

13

YOUR PERSONAL
ACTION PLAN

The constant interplay of hormones within your body is an amazing and complex process, but the key to harmony boils down to a relatively simple set of actions. You could think of these as a personal path, tailored to your own needs, which will enable you to achieve and maintain a state of balance. The journey begins with identifying the specific elements of your own life that are contributing to or detracting from a state of hormonal harmony.

Because you are a unique individual, your needs, strengths and weaknesses will also be unique. To help set your own priorities, consider the key areas below, which were covered in more detail in the previous chapters, and use the *Hormone Harmony Habits Checklist* at the end of this chapter to track your progress.

FOOD BASICS

It's difficult to change eating habits, and most people don't feel the need to do so. In a survey by the American Dietetic Association, 79 percent of respondents were satisfied with the way they eat, but that doesn't mean most people are eating in a way that supports hormonal balance or an optimum level of well-being.

Refined carbohydrates, rich in sugar and/or starch, cause rapid spikes in blood sugar. These, in turn, trigger hormonal imbalance, promote food cravings for more sugary and starchy foods, contribute to weight gain and increase risks for diabetes, heart disease and cancer. In contrast, fresh vegetables, lean proteins, healthy fats and a moderate amount of high-fiber fruit maintain stable levels of blood sugar and promote hormonal balance. Small, frequent meals or snacks are most effective in managing blood sugar and sustaining healthy levels of energy.

To see if your personal eating habits can be improved, consider these key questions.

- Do you get cravings for starchy or sugary foods, such as cookies, candy, cakes, buns, french fries, creamy mashed potatoes or sugary sodas (regular or diet)?
- Do you get ravenously hungry to the point where you just grab whatever you can?
- Do you hit a wall midafternoon when you run out of energy and can't think straight?
- Are you gaining weight for no apparent reason?
- Are you experiencing hot flashes?
- Are your moods unpredictable?
- Are you exhausted when you wake up in the morning?

If you answer "yes" to one or more of the questions above, there's room for improvement in your eating habits. While food is only one aspect of lifestyle, it is as basic as can be. We have to eat, and what we ingest can work for or against us. To start making improvements, look over the summary of key food habits below and pick one that you can start to implement right away. After that practice becomes routine, implement a second one, make it a habit, and then adopt a third one, and so on. By making gradual changes, it's possible to transform your habits gradually rather than making a heroic effort to change everything at once, backsliding, trying again, backsliding, and getting into a vicious no-win cycle.

EAT BREAKFAST. If you like cereal, choose one made with 100 percent whole grain and without added sugar. Traditional oatmeal is a good choice. For some additional protein, add a small protein drink. Or eat eggs–preferably cooked with little or no butter–with whole grain toast. If you like a hot beverage in the morning, green tea is a good choice, but coffee is fine too, as long as you aren't sensitive to the caffeine. Drinking soda for breakfast is the worst way to start the day.

HAVE A MIDMORNING SNACK if you eat lunch more than three or four hours after breakfast, but one without candy, cookies, doughnuts, chips or other refined foods. A small handful of raw almonds, or an organic apple or pear—with a small piece of low-fat cheese if you prefer—are good choices.

REPLACE SODA, at any time of day, with green tea, other herbal tea or water. If this seems impossible, start by eliminating the soda you drink during the earlier part of the day. Decrease your intake gradually, until soda is out of your life.

FOR LUNCH, eat approximately 2 to 3 ounces of organic poultry or fish and as many non-starchy vegetables as you like. Non-starchy vegetables are one type of food you can eat in unlimited quantities–as long as they aren't fried, accompanied by butter or covered in high-fat creamy dressings or sauces. To add flavor, try different seasonings and a little extra virgin olive oil or a low-fat or non-fat dressing (without artificial ingredients) that appeals to your taste buds. Dip vegetables lightly in dressing. Beans or whole grains will give you some additional nutrients and fiber. Key things to avoid: any type of processed or cured meats, which usually contain chemical additives and increase risk for cancer. These include hot dogs, smoked meats and packaged luncheon meats, including ham and turkey. Uncured sliced meats, such as turkey and ham, without any artificial ingredients are available in natural-food supermarkets, but check ingredients carefully to make sure they don't contain artificial smoke flavoring or nitrates.

HAVE A MIDAFTERNOON SNACK similar to your mid-morning snack. Any type of raw nuts will work; dry roast-ed ones are second-best. Or, if you have leftovers from lunch, they can make an excellent snack. If you buy lunch, the portion of meat will usually be larger than 2 to 3 ounces, and your body will function better if you save some for midafternoon, rather than eating it all at lunchtime.

FOR DINNER, eat another 2 to 3 ounces of fish or organic poultry, or occasionally, organic lean red meat (hormone-free is second best), with non-starchy vegetables and whole grains or legumes. If you can't prepare food from scratch, look for organic frozen meals and add more vegetables, or find take-out food that is prepared without batter, grilled rather than fried, and preferably organic.

IF YOU LIKE DESSERT, consider fruit, a small piece of dark chocolate or a low-calorie pudding made without artificial additives. If you eat well all day long, it shouldn't be too difficult to control what you eat by this time of day, and a small treat (size really matters) isn't likely to do damage.

IF YOU NEED A SNACK BEFORE GOING TO BED, follow the same principles as for snacks earlier in the day.

If you're away from home much of the day, finding healthy meals and snacks can be challenging. One solution is to take food with you. Another is to do a little sleuthing and find some restaurants with healthy options, or stores with good quality take-out. Once your body starts getting used to eating additive-free, clean food, you will quickly be able to gauge the quality of prepared food from any establishment, even if you don't have a complete list of ingredients. The key thing to look for is fresh ingredients, cooked in a way that brings out natural flavors, rather than batters and sauces that mask poor-quality food.

As a general rule, the importance of vegetables can't be overstated. For overall health, including reducing risk for cancer, adults should eat at least 14 ounces of non-starchy vegetables and fruit each day. That's almost a pound, so it may sound like a lot, but it isn't. For example, one-half of a medium bell pepper (green, red, orange or yellow) weighs about 3 ounces; one medium tomato weighs about 4.5 ounces; 10 stalks of steamed baby asparagus about 3 ounces; and one small apple or half a medium pear weigh about 4 to 5 ounces. Combined, with either the apple or the half-pear, these choices would total just over 14 ounces.

It's not surprising if you think this seems like a lot of vegetables and fruit in one day; culturally, we underestimate the value of these kinds of foods. For instance, in some restaurants, if you ask for tomato instead of hash browns with breakfast, you might get only one or two slices because the tomato is mistakenly viewed as a garnish. Bottom line: If at least 14 ounces of nature's best seems unrealistic, then it may be time to adopt a new perspective.

If you embrace the style of eating described above, you don't have to feel deprived. If you're going out for dinner on the weekend, enjoy yourself. Don't feel guilty about eating whatever you want or having a drink, in moderation. Your body will be in good shape as a result of being fed well all week, and one meal isn't likely to ruin everything. In fact, you're more likely to stay on a healthy path by giving yourself a treat once a week. And, you may be the only person at your table who is truly enjoying a treat, without the guilt we so often see people expressing on special occasions.

STRESS CONTROL

Stress increases our production of cortisol and, when it becomes chronic, disrupts balance among hormones. To start reducing your ongoing stress load each day, give yourself a recess, even if only for a few minutes. Use that time to "smell the roses," in whatever way works for you, whether it's walking around the block, sitting on a park bench, taking a few deep breaths, doing a crossword puzzle—or literally enjoying the fragrance of some flowers.

"No time" is the most common excuse for not taking some time to ourselves, but it isn't a good one. Stepping aside from whatever is going on in your day puts you in a better position to deal more effectively with irritating people and challenging situations and can help you to manage your schedule from a position of strength rather than weakness. If you feel really strapped for time, pretend you have to brush your teeth an extra time but instead of grabbing a toothbrush, give yourself a recess. And try taking a "wet towel" approach, setting boundaries and other suggestions outlined in chapter 6.

TOXIN REDUCTION

Choosing organic foods whenever possible, especially for your staples, will significantly reduce the stress of toxins in your body. Because you purchase food frequently, start looking for organic versions of the usual things on your grocery list the next time you shop. And when you have to replace soaps, laundry and household-cleaning products, choose fragrance-free, non-toxic varieties without antibacterial ingredients. Meanwhile, get rid of any air fresheners with "fragrance" and keep your home well ventilated. For more ways to reduce your toxic load, look over chapter 7.

CORRECT EXERCISE

Ultimately, we all need regular aerobic and strength training to maintain muscle, bone mass and overall fitness. However, depending on your starting point, you may need gentler forms of exercise at the beginning, such as those described in chapter 6. Brisk walking is a simple way to start getting some aerobic exercise, and chapter 8 includes a basic strength-training routine. The most important thing is to do a level and type of activity that reduces stress and helps to restore balance, rather than pushing too hard too fast, which will increase stress and hormonal disruption.

NUTRITIONAL INSURANCE

A good quality multivitamin, CoQ10 and fish oil will provide nutritional insurance, help to counteract stress and support stable levels of blood sugar and energy. Together, these elements will make it easier to control appetite and weight and to ward off triggers of hormonal imbalance. Additional nutritional supplements, covered in chapter 10, may help in specific situations.

BIOIDENTICAL HORMONES

By maintaining a healthy lifestyle, many women can achieve and maintain a state of well-being. However, if you develop the habits that support healthy hormone balance but continue to experience uncomfortable or debilitating symptoms, it's wise to seek out a qualified medical doctor who can take a look at your personal situation, obtain appropriate tests, and give you a personalized program to address your needs. In such a situation, the physician should clearly understand and respect your goals and work with you to bring about the results you seek.

THE BOTTOM LINE

Even though the factors that promote hormonal harmony are universal, your personal circumstances are unique. What worked for a friend or relative may or may not produce the same result for you, and vice versa. In assessing your own situation, be honest. If you love drinking soda throughout the day and discount the fact that it could be affecting the way your body functions, you aren't doing yourself a favor. Make an effort to substitute healthier beverages, especially with breakfast. Giving your body a good foundation in the morning will make it easier to manage food and drinks later in the day. Or, if you love fast food, recognize that immediate gratification is its only benefit; once it goes down your throat, it works against you.

Changing long-term habits can be difficult, but it isn't impossible. Many women have succeeded in removing soda, fast food, candy, cookies, chips or other unhealthy favorites from their daily routines. And once they took that step, they discovered it's not too difficult to maintain a healthier way of life because they have never felt so good, even when they were much younger. The trick is to make sufficient changes to experience the benefits, and you, too, may never want to look back.

The *Hormone Harmony Habits Checklist* on the next two pages will help you to start making changes and to track your progress.

HORMONE HARMONY HABITS CHECKLIST

Develop these habits, one by one, to bring about hormonal harmony. Make copies of these two pages or download and print a one-page version from **www.hormoneharmony.org/checklist** and each day, check off habits you have adopted or maintained. For more tools to enhance your life, see *How to Track Your Progress* in the Appendix.

Week starting Sunday ___(month)___ ___(day)___ ___(year)___	SUNDAY	MONDAY	TUESDAY	WEDNESDAY	THURSDAY	FRIDAY	SATURDAY
Give yourself a recess at least once a day.							
Drink filtered water and green or other herbal tea instead of soda.							
Stay away from sugary and/or starchy foods, especially in the mornings and after dinner.							
Eat small meals frequently, with ample vegetables, lean protein, whole grains and legumes, and some raw nuts and fresh fruit.							

Choose organic versions of your staple foods and beverages, and others as much as possible.						
Keep your home well ventilated and avoid air fresheners with "fragrance."						
Avoid synthetic fragrance and antibacterial ingredients in soaps, beauty, grooming, laundry and household-cleaning products.						
Engage in enough physical activity, of the right type, for your body.						
Take a good quality multivitamin, CoQ10 and fish oil.						
If necessary, take additional supplements for specific situations.						
If the above actions don't bring about a state of well-being, locate and consult a medical doctor who has specialized training in nutrition, fitness and bioidentical hormone replacement therapy (BHRT), to define your personal path to optimum health.						

14

HORMONE HARMONY
FOR MEN

In recent years, testosterone levels among American men have been declining substantially, beyond what is normal as a function of aging. In addition to endowing male characteristics, testosterone is considered the "life force hormone." It supports sex drive and sexual function, helps to maintain lean muscle mass, protects against bone loss and is associated with aggression. In studies of men, low levels of testosterone have been associated with depression, heart disease, diabetes, Alzheimer's disease and prostate cancer.

Although testosterone levels do drop naturally as men get older, we are now facing a new situation, where levels of the hormone are decreasing prematurely among men in their late 30s and 40s, and decreasing more intensely than nature intended among many older men. Why is this happening? It's a symptom of our way of life. Does this mean all men should automatically receive testosterone therapy? No, but it does mean that improvements in nutrition, stress management and exercise and reductions in exposure to everyday toxins will benefit most—if not all—men. In some situations, some degree of hormone therapy may also be beneficial, but even then lifestyle factors are critical. Hormone therapy is not a substitute for a healthy diet, stress reduction and physical activity.

TESTOSTERONE ROBBERS

At the New England Research Institutes in Boston, a number of studies have examined some connections between levels of testosterone, lifestyle and men's quality of life. These are some of the findings.

- A large waist is the most important contributor to low testosterone levels and non-optimum symptoms, including low sex drive, erectile dysfunction, osteoporosis, sleep disturbances, depressed mood, lethargy and diminished physical performance. According to the study, which examined data on more than 1,800 men, testosterone levels also correlate with overall state of health. Men in excellent health are most likely to have higher levels of testosterone and least likely to experience non-optimum symptoms.
- Weight gain accelerates decline in testosterone levels. According to a study that tracked more than 1,600 men for up to 17 years, an increase in body mass index (BMI) of 4 to 5 points is comparable to 10 years of aging, in terms of testosterone decline. BMI is an indicator of whether a person is overweight, obese or at a healthy weight. As an example, for a man who is 5 feet 11 inches tall, an increase in weight from 180 to 207 pounds would be a 4-point jump in BMI. The loss of a spouse triggers a similar accelerated decline in testosterone levels.
- For many men, erectile dysfunction can be resolved with weight loss, instead of medications, according to a study of 401 men. Smoking and overall poor health

increase risk for the condition. Since ED is associated with heart disease, the researchers concluded that treating the condition with lifestyle changes, rather than medication, could produce far-reaching benefits for men's overall health. (To check your own BMI, see the chart on the next two pages.)

CULTURAL STEREOTYPES

The typical Western lifestyle promotes a large waist and overall weight gain, intensifying natural hormonal fluctuations and speeding up the decline of testosterone and the aging process. Contrary to marketing campaigns, eating fast food and drinking giant tubs of soda doesn't make a "real man." In fact, greasy burgers, fries and sugary or starchy refined foods, combined with chronic stress and too many TV channels, trigger hormonal disruption, which—to put it bluntly—deprives a guy of his manhood.

Cultural stereotypes can also act as a deterrent to better health, because men are generally expected to ignore physical discomfort and "suck it up," rather than taking steps to address the root of a problem. Magazines, web sites and books that target women have been talking about "well-being" for years, but no comparable term has gained popularity in male-oriented media. Nevertheless, there is no rational reason why well-being, or optimum health, should be limited to any one gender.

Any man can experience one or more symptoms of hormonal disruption occasionally, but if the situation becomes bothersome, or worse, significantly affects day-to-day life, it needs attention. Men and women are equally eligible to be in the best

BODY MASS INDEX

Medically speaking, Body Mass Index (BMI) is used to determine if an individual is underweight, in a healthy range, over-weight or obese. Health risks increase in the overweight range and increase further with obesity.

Locate your height in the left-hand column, then your weight. Your BMI will be at the top of your weight column. BMI may not accurately reflect health status for a minority of people who are very lean and exceptionally muscular but for most people, this is what BMI numbers indicate:

Underweight = less than 18.5   Normal weight = 18.5-24.9   Overweight = 25-29.9   Obesity = 30 or greater

BMI	19	20	21	22	23	24	25	26	27	28	29	30	31	32	33	34	35
Height (inches)								Body Weight (pounds)									
58	91	96	100	105	110	115	119	124	129	134	138	143	148	153	158	162	167
59	94	99	104	109	114	119	124	128	133	138	143	148	153	158	163	168	173
60	97	102	107	112	118	123	128	133	138	143	148	153	158	163	168	174	179
61	100	106	111	116	122	127	132	137	143	148	153	158	164	169	174	180	185
62	104	109	115	120	126	131	136	142	147	153	158	164	169	175	180	186	191
63	107	113	118	124	130	135	141	146	152	158	163	169	175	180	186	191	197

BMI	19	20	21	22	23	24	25	26	27	28	29	30	31	32	33	34	35
Height (inches)							Body Weight (pounds)										
64	110	116	122	128	134	140	145	151	157	163	169	174	180	186	192	197	204
65	114	120	126	132	138	144	150	156	162	168	174	180	186	192	198	204	210
66	118	124	130	136	142	148	155	161	167	173	179	186	192	198	204	210	216
67	121	127	134	140	146	153	159	166	172	178	185	191	198	204	211	217	223
68	125	131	138	144	151	158	164	171	177	184	190	197	203	210	216	223	230
69	128	135	142	149	155	162	169	176	182	189	196	203	209	216	223	230	236
70	132	139	146	153	160	167	174	181	188	195	202	209	216	222	229	236	243
71	136	143	150	157	165	172	179	186	193	200	208	215	222	229	236	243	250
72	140	147	154	162	169	177	184	191	199	206	213	221	228	235	242	250	258
73	144	151	159	166	174	182	189	197	204	212	219	227	235	242	250	257	265
74	148	155	163	171	179	186	194	202	210	218	225	233	241	249	256	264	272
75	152	160	168	176	184	192	200	208	216	224	232	240	248	256	264	272	279
76	156	164	172	180	189	197	205	213	221	230	238	246	254	263	271	279	287

For BMI above 35, visit the National Heart, Lung and Blood Institute at www.nhlbi.nih.gov/guidelines/obesity/bmi_tbl2.htm.

SYMPTOMS OF HORMONAL DISRUPTION

Non-optimum levels of testosterone, cortisol, insulin, thyroid and/or other hormones may produce a variety of symptoms, including:

- Aches and pains
- Allergies
- Breast enlargement
- Constipation
- Difficulty losing weight
- Erectile dysfunction
- Feeling apathetic or depressed
- Feeling lethargic, exhausted or burned out
- Frequent trips to the bathroom
- Frequently feeling cold
- Headaches
- Infertility
- Insomnia or interrupted sleep
- Irritability
- Lack of motivation
- Low sex drive
- Mental fog
- More frequent colds and flu
- Muscles shrinking and body fat increasing
- Oily skin
- Poor concentration
- Prostate problems
- Sleep apnea
- Snoring louder, longer or more frequently
- Weight gain, especially in the belly

shape possible, and both sexes deserve to achieve such a state. And, despite some obvious hormonal differences, both require the same basic lifestyle approaches to restore balance. These include: Eating a diet with little or no refined food rich in sugary and/or starchy carbohydrates, managing stress, avoiding exposure to everyday toxins, getting the right type of exercise and obtaining some nutritional insurance from key dietary supplements. In some situations, bioidentical hormones may also be beneficial, but they should not be viewed as a magic cure-all or a substitute for a healthy way of life.

STRESS, MEN AND HORMONES

When we think of men and hormones, testosterone is the one that most often comes to mind, but no single hormone works alone. Rather, there is a constant interplay of many hormones in our bodies, and the key to optimum health is balance among these. Hormones work together like a football team, and an injury to one player can upset every strategy in a coach's playbook.

This is the most common way in which hormones malfunction in a man's body: Chronic stress, due to life circumstances and/or poor diet, triggers production of too much cortisol, the "fight or flight" hormone. This, in turn, sets off a chain reaction that leads to depressed levels of testosterone, resulting in the types of symptoms listed above. In the simplest terms, this sequence of events reduces a guy's manhood to a greater degree than the natural aging process.

Let's take a more detailed look at what happens in this kind of chain reaction.

- The human body uses the same building blocks to make cortisol and testosterone; in a healthy state, both hormones are produced in balanced amounts. However, when stress creates excessive demand for cortisol, too many building blocks are used to manufacture it, and testosterone production suffers. In other words, the raw materials to make testosterone are diverted to produce cortisol.

- Over time, elevated levels of cortisol lead to increased belly fat, and this fat contains an enzyme (aromatase) that encourages testosterone to be converted into estrogen, further reducing levels of testosterone. And, while men require and naturally produce some estrogen, when levels of this hormone are too high, they negate the effects of whatever testosterone is present, contributing to weight gain, breast enlargement, sexual problems and other symptoms.

Ironically, short bursts of stress increase production of testosterone, as well as cortisol. However, ongoing stress, which is prevalent today, depletes testosterone. Other factors, such as illness, use of performance-enhancing drugs earlier in life and some medical treatments, such as chemotherapy and, for some men, cholesterol-lowering medications, can disrupt hormones. However, the lifestyle situation described above is the most prevalent culprit.

DIETARY STRESS TRIGGERS

Relationships at home or work, financial pressures and career challenges are among common triggers of stress, but diet is another one which is usually ignored. Eating the wrong types of food is much like pumping regular unleaded, instead of premium fuel into a Ferrari. In a man's body, the wrong fuel can cause elevated cortisol levels and bring about a state of chronic stress. In addition, diet-induced stress will magnify the physical impact of stressful life situations. In contrast, the right foods can buffer against damage from the strains of life and help to restore and support a guy's internal engine so that he can be on top of his game.

The wrong foods are sugary and starchy ones, and sugary beverages such as soda. After we eat carbohydrates, they are converted into blood sugar, a form of fuel that can be used by cells to produce energy. The hormone insulin is secreted to deliver the fuel to cells. Foods that are rich in sugar and/or starch convert very rapidly, causing a sudden upward spike in blood sugar, and insulin then has to deliver a large supply of fuel in a very short period of time. There are three negative consequences to this scenario.

1. The spike in blood sugar is a form of physical stress that triggers excess production of cortisol.
2. Over time, as muscle cells are repeatedly overwhelmed with extra-large amounts of blood sugar, they stop accepting it. So, instead of being burned as energy, the fuel is delivered to fat cells for storage, causing weight gain, especially in the belly. And belly fat promotes production of cortisol. (The phenomena of muscle cells refusing to accept blood glucose is known as insulin resistance, and is covered in more detail in chapter 2.)

3. This cycle is self-perpetuating because, after rapidly spiking upward, blood-sugar levels crash to below-normal levels, causing cravings for more sugary, starchy foods or sugary drinks, leading to more diet-induced stress.

How does this relate to greasy burgers and fries? The fries are high in starch. The burgers come with starchy buns made with refined flour. In addition, large amounts of saturated fat in such meals make it more difficult for these carbohydrates to be burned efficiently to produce energy, so more calories end up being stored as fat. To add insult to injury, burgers and fries are usually accompanied by large sodas that contain large amounts of sugar. Diet sodas with zero-calorie sweeteners don't solve the problem. While technically sugar-free, diet drinks may trick the brain into stimulating appetite because when we ingest something sweet, our bodies expect calories. All sugary foods, mashed potatoes, chips and other starchy foods do the same type of damage. Aim to replace these hormone-disrupting foods with lean protein and plenty of non-starchy vegetables at each meal, as well as high-fiber fruits such as apples, pears and berries as desserts or snacks.

The interplay between food, insulin and cortisol is described more extensively in chapter 2. That chapter is applicable to men as well as women with one difference: For men, the major liability of elevated cortisol is the cycle that leads to low levels of testosterone, as described above, whereas for women, low levels of progesterone are the most common result of a poor diet.

Chronic high demand for cortisol, which is produced by the adrenal glands, can also interfere with the function of the thyroid, which drives metabolism. Low levels of thyroid hormone are also common, affecting as many as one in seven adults. Where there is a malfunction in the adrenal glands as well as a thyroid problem, if the thyroid is treated without addressing adrenal issues, a person can feel worse.

OTHER LIFESTYLE ISSUES

Several key lifestyle factors will help to get and keep your levels of testosterone and other hormones at healthy levels.

PHYSICAL ACTIVITY

Stress can also be induced by the wrong type of exercise, too much exercise, or too little recovery time between workouts. On the other hand, physical activity that is the right intensity for your personal fitness level will help to reduce stress as well as improve the health of your heart and counteract age-related loss of muscle. To get the full benefits, you need regular aerobic exercise for the heart and two strength-training sessions per week, working all the major muscle groups. If you do extensive exercise and find yourself exhausted much of the time, you could be overdoing it.

For any man who currently gets no regular exercise, it's time to start. Walking is one simple option. Another approach is to revive your participation in a sport you once enjoyed. Keep in mind that you have to start slow and work up to higher levels of performance and give your body time to recover in between bouts. To reduce stress, choose physical activities you enjoy doing. And, get adequate sleep.

SLEEP

Getting enough restful sleep is a prerequisite for maintaining optimum testosterone production, preventing cortisol levels from rising too high and supporting efficient burning of food as fuel. Good ways to improve your sleep include allowing enough time for eight hours of rest and relaxing by doing something other than watching TV or using a computer before going to bed, as both activities tend to increase stress levels.

Disrupted hormones can interfere with restful sleep in both men and women, but the underlying hormonal mechanisms are different. Among men, low testosterone, malfunctioning cortisol or a combination of the two can cause sleep apnea, which occurs in approximately 9 percent of men and is more common among those who are obese. When this occurs, in addition to snoring, there is a repeated difficulty or interruption in breathing, which disrupts sleep. A vicious cycle occurs because lack of sleep leads to elevated cortisol, lower levels of testosterone and more sleep problems. Controlling stress and weight are basic strategies to reverse the situation.

STRESS CONTROL

In addition to reducing natural testosterone production, chronic stress promotes weight gain. To reduce stress, the key thing is to find something that works for you. Some people relax by doing solitary activities, which could be running, hiking, shooting hoops, reading or building things. Others hate being alone and relax by spending time with friends, playing a team sport or a game of cards. The important point is that human beings need a break from the usual routines and demands of day-to-day life.

That break could be something as simple as turning off your cell phone while driving and listening to your favorite music, with the volume set as high, or low, as you like. Just remember to give yourself a break.

TOXIN REDUCTION

One of the ways toxins damage our bodies is by disrupting hormones, and you can exert some control over your own exposure. Pesticides and chemical additives in foods are one of the major sources of pollution for our bodies and can be reduced by eating organic foods and those without artificial ingredients. Personal grooming products are another common source of toxins. The key types of ingredients to avoid are synthetic fragrance, usually listed as "fragrance" or "scent" on most products, and antibacterial ingredients. Air fresheners and laundry and home cleaning products with the same ingredients should also be avoided.

DIETARY SUPPLEMENTS

A good quality multivitamin provides nutritional insurance. In addition, fish oil supports overall health, including the heart, and may help to keep the prostate healthy. Studies have found that regularly eating fish or taking fish oil supplements may improve prostate cancer survival. And, for any man over 35, CoQ10 is also advisable. Chapter 9 provides more detailed information about these. Some additional dietary supplements contain a combination of nutrients to support healthy testosterone levels and prostate health, and some of the companies that make these types of formulas are listed in *Supplement Sources* in the Appendix.

SAW PALMETTO

Long before Western medicine existed in the New World, Native Americans used berries of the saw palmetto plant to treat men's urinary tract problems and to boost libido. Today, saw palmetto is available as a dietary supplement and is most often used to prevent or relieve symptoms of a non-cancerous enlarged prostate, or benign prostatic hyperplasia (BPH). Although research results are mixed, it appears that the herb may prevent growth of the prostate as men age, thereby helping to avoid or alleviate urinary problems resulting from an enlarged prostate. In men's formulas, saw palmetto is often combined with an extract of nettle root because the two herbs may work synergistically.

BIOIDENTICAL HORMONES

If you suspect your testosterone levels may be below optimum, the first step is to make lifestyle changes. If that doesn't resolve the situation, or if symptoms are too severe to wait, you can consult a physician who has specialized training in treating hormone imbalances with bioidentical hormones. Chapters 11 and 12 describe bioidentical hormone therapy in some detail. Although some of that information specifically addresses women's issues, the underlying concepts are not gender specific. A qualified medical doctor should do tests to get an overall picture of your hormone status, gather information about your symptoms and medical history and give you a program that encompasses necessary lifestyle changes—including nutrition, fitness and stress management—as well as prescribing any hormone treatment.

LIFESTYLE SNAPSHOT

Among men and women, the same lifestyle factors drive up cortisol, disrupt hormones and accelerate the aging process. In addition to diet, these include stressful life situations, exposure to toxins and the wrong types of exercise. Chapters 2 through 9 cover these aspects in more detail, and chapter 13 gives an overview, tips on where to start and a checklist to monitor progress. These can be used as a guide for men as well as women.

While the basics of a lifestyle that keeps hormones synchronized are not gender specific, culturally, men face their own obstacles. For example, healthy food choices may elicit a variety of responses, depending on where you live and the company you keep. In some circles, if you're ordering lunch with a group of guys, steaks or burgers, fries and soda may be the popular menu choices. Choosing a salad with grilled fish or some other type of lean protein and drinking mineral water or iced tea may provoke some derogatory comments or jokes. On the other hand, if you're in health-oriented circles, the steak and fries may provoke some odd looks.

Chances are, unless your friends and co-workers are in exceptional physical condition, you may well find yourself oddly alone in adopting healthy lifestyle habits. But don't be discouraged. If those around you can't see the wisdom of living in good health right now, perhaps they will come around in the future. Meanwhile, you can enjoy the benefits of being in better shape.

APPENDIX

HOW TO FIND QUALIFIED PHYSICIANS

BodyLogicMD
www.BodyLogicMD.com
Visit the web site to locate physicians throughout the United States who specialize in bioidentical hormones, nutrition and fitness. BodyLogicMD is a network of independent medical practices owned by doctors who meet specific educational requirements and participate in continuing education to stay abreast of the latest science regarding bioidentical hormone therapy, nutrition and fitness.

If you cannot find a BodyLogicMD physician in your vicinity, the compounding pharmacies below may help you identify some physicians in your area that are qualified to provide bioidentical hormone replacement therapy.

COMPOUNDING PHARMACIES

Bioidentical hormones require a prescription from a licensed physician; pharmacies do not issue prescriptions. The pharmacies below can fill prescriptions throughout the United States and accept payment from many health plans. They can help you determine if your health insurance will pay for hormone preparations prescribed by your doctor and, where appropriate, assist you in obtaining reimbursement from your insurance provider.

Medaus
www.medaus.com

University Compounding Pharmacy
www.ucprx.com

LABORATORY TESTING SOURCES

These labs provide testing services for physicians throughout the United States. A physician will determine the most appropriate tests, based upon a patient's health history, recent medical tests and current situation.

LAB	TYPES OF TESTS	METHOD
ZRT Laboratory www.zrtlabs.com	hormone	saliva, blood spot, urine
Genova Diagnostics www.genovadiagnostics.com	hormone	saliva, urine
Quest Diagnostics www.questdiagnostics.com	hormone	blood
NeuroScience www.neurorelief.com	neurotransmitter hormone	saliva, blood, urine
ALCAT www.alcat.com	food sensitivities food allergies	blood
SpectraCell Laboratories www.spectracell.com	nutrient levels	blood

BIOIDENTICAL HORMONE BRANDS

Some mass-produced bioidentical hormone brands that are available by prescription from any pharmacy are listed below. As the book went to press, there were no mass-produced combinations of estrogen and progesterone that contained bioidentical forms of both hormones. For updates, visit www.hormoneharmony.org.

BIOIDENTICAL ESTROGEN

PATCH: Alora, Climara, Esclim, Estraderm, Vivelle

TOPICAL GEL: EstroGel

TOPICAL CREAM: Estrasorb

VAGINAL CREAM: Estrace

VAGINAL RING: Estring, Femring

VAGINAL TABLET: Vagifem

PILL: Estrace

BIOIDENTICAL PROGESTERONE*

PILL: Prometrium (not recommended for anyone with peanut allergies)

VAGINAL GEL: Prochieve 4%

BIOIDENTICAL TESTOSTERONE

TOPICAL GEL: AndroGel

---

*For optimum benefits, many women require prescription-strength bioidentical progesterone in a topical gel or cream. As this book went to press, there was no such mass-produced product available in the United States.

SUPPLEMENT SOURCES

The brands below are available from licensed health professionals. As the book went to press, each web site with an asterisk (*) offered an online locator to help you find practitioners in your area who carry the company's products.

Biotics Research Corporation www.bioticsresearch.com	**Ortho Molecular Products** www.orthomolecularproducts.com*
Future Formulations, LLC www.futureformulations.com*	**Pharmax LLC** www.pharmaxllc.com
Metagenics www.metagenics.com*	**Xymogen** www.xymogen.com

HOW TO TRACK YOUR PROGRESS

Keeping track of lifestyle changes will help you take control of your health. The *Hormone Harmony Habits Checklist*, at the end of chapter 13, will help you get started. For convenience, visit www.hormoneharmony.org/checklist to download and print copies of the checklist. Make a note of this web page. Anyone can visit the Hormone Harmony web site but the page containing the checklist cannot be accessed from the main site, as it is designed specifically for readers of this book.

More tools are being developed to help you manage your life and health care, and to keep your hormones in optimum balance. If you would like to preview these before they are released to the general public, and to receive ongoing tips from Dr. Stanton, sign up for alerts at www.hormoneharmony.org.

SELECTED REFERENCES

CHAPTER I

Barclay AW, Petocz P, McMillan-Price J, Flood VM, Prvan T, Mitchell P, Brand-Miller JC. Glycemic index, glycemic load, and chronic disease risk–a meta-analysis of observational studies. *American Journal of Clinical Nutrition.* 2008 Mar;87(3):627-37.

Brand-Miller J, Dickinson S, Barclay A, Celermajer D. The glycemic index and cardiovascular disease risk. *Current Atherosclerosis Reports.* 2007 Dec;9(6):479-85.

Critser G. *Fat Land.* New York, NY: Houghton Mifflin, 2003.

Curtis BM, O'Keefe JH Jr. Autonomic tone as a cardiovascular risk factor: the dangers of chronic fight or flight. *Mayo Clinic Proceedings.* 2002 Jan;77(1):45-54.

Kopp W. Chronically increased activity of the sympathetic nervous system: our diet-related "evolutionary" inheritance. *The Journal of Nutrition, Health & Aging.* 2009 Jan;13(1):27-9.

Kopp W. The atherogenic potential of dietary carbohydrate. *Preventive Medicine.* 2007 Jan; 44(1):82-4.

Nestle M. *Food Politics.* Berkeley, CA: University of California Press, 2002.

Schlosser E. *Fast Food Nation.* New York, NY: Harper Perennial, 2005.

Suter PM. Carbohydrates and dietary fiber. *Handbook of Experimental Pharmacology.* 2005;(170):231-61.

Wansink B. *Marketing Nutrition.* Chicago, IL: University of Illinois Press, 2005.

Wright JV. Bio-identical steroid hormone replacement: selected observations from 23 years of clinical and laboratory practice. *Annals of the New York Academy of Sciences.* 2005 Dec;1057:506-24.

Wu T, Dorn JP, Donahue RP, Sempos CT, Trevisan M. Associations of serum C-reactive protein with fasting insulin, glucose, and glycosylated hemoglobin: the Third National Health and Nutrition

Examination Survey, 1988-1994. *American Journal of Epidemiology.* 2002 Jan 1;155(1):65-71.

CHAPTER 2

Campfield LA, Smith FJ, Rosenbaum M, Hirsch J. Human eating: evidence for a physiological basis using a modified paradigm. *Neuroscience and Biobehavioral Reviews.*1996;20(1):133-7.

Huerta R, Mena A, Malacara JM, de León JD. Symptoms at the menopausal and premenopausal years: their relationship with insulin, glucose, cortisol, FSH, prolactin, obesity and attitudes towards sexuality. *Psychoneuroendocrinology.* 1995;20(8):851-64.

Kronenberg HM (Editor), Melmed S (Editor), Polonsky KS (Editor), Reed Larsen P (Editor). *Williams Textbook of Endocrinology,* 11th Ed. Philadelphia, PA: Saunders, 2007.

La Berge AF. How the ideology of low fat conquered America. *Journal of the History of Medicine and Allied Sciences.* 2008 Apr;63(2): 139-77.

Ludwig DS. Dietary Glycemic Index and Obesity. *Journal of Nutrition.* 2000;130:280S-283S.

Malacara JM, Huerta R, Rivera B, Esparza S, Fajardo ME. Menopause in normal and uncomplicated NIDDM women: physical and emotional symptoms and hormone profile. *Maturitas.* 1997 Sep;28(1): 35-45.

Rodin J, Wack J, Ferrannini E, DeFronzo RA. Effect of insulin and glucose on feeding behavior. *Metabolism.* 1985 Sep;34(9):826-31.

Sabia S, Fournier A, Mesrine S, Boutron-Ruault MC, Clavel-Chapelon F. Risk factors for onset of menopausal symptoms: results from a large cohort study. *Maturitas.* 2008 Jun 20;60(2):108-21.

Thompson DA, Campbell RG. Hunger in humans induced by 2-deoxy-D-glucose: glucoprivic control of taste preference and food intake. *Science.* 1977 Dec 9;198(4321):1065-8.

White PD. The tardy growth of preventive cardiology. *American Journal of Cardioliology.* 1972 Jun;29(6):886-8.

CHAPTER 3

Augustin LS, Polesel J, Bosetti C, Kendall CW, La Vecchia C, Parpinel M, Conti E, Montella M, Franceschi S, Jenkins DJ, Dal Maso L. Dietary glycemic index, glycemic load and ovarian cancer risk: a case-control study in Italy. *Annals of Oncology.* 2003 Jan;14(1):78-84.

Brand-Miller J, Foster-Powell K. *The New Glucose Revolution Shopper's Guide to GI Values 2009.* Cambridge, MA: De Capo Life Long, 2009.

Folsom AR, Demissie Z, Harnack L; Iowa Women's Health Study. Glycemic index, glycemic load, and incidence of endometrial cancer: the Iowa women's health study. *Nutrition and Cancer.* 2003;46(2): 119-24.

Kaaja RJ. Metabolic syndrome and the menopause. *Menopause International.* 2008 Mar;14(1):21-5.

Lajous M, Boutron-Ruault MC, Fabre A, Clavel-Chapelon F, Romieu I. Carbohydrate intake, glycemic index, glycemic load, and risk of postmenopausal breast cancer in a prospective study of French women. *American Journal of Clinical Nutrition.* 2008 May;87(5): 1384-91.

Lajous M, Willett W, Lazcano-Ponce E, Sanchez-Zamorano LM, Hernandez-Avila M, Romieu I. Glycemic load, glycemic index, and the risk of breast cancer among Mexican women. *Cancer Causes Control.* 2005 Dec;16(10):1165-9.

Lieberman, S. *Transitions Lifestyle System Easy-to-Use Glycemic Index Food Guide.* Garden City Park, NY: Square One Publishers, 2006.

Ludwig DS. The glycemic index: physiological mechanisms relating to obesity, diabetes, and cardiovascular disease. *Journal of the American Medical Association.* 2002 May 8;287(18):2414-23.

McCann SE, McCann WE, Hong CC, Marshall JR, Edge SB, Trevisan M, Muti P, Freudenheim JL. Dietary patterns related to glycemic index and load and risk of premenopausal and post-menopausal breast cancer in the Western New York Exposure and Breast Cancer Study. *American Journal of Clinical Nutrition.* 2007 Aug;86(2):465-71.

Official Website of the Glycemic Index and GI Database. www.glycemicindex.com.

Sieri S, Pala V, Brighenti F, Pellegrini N, Muti P, Micheli A, Evangelista A, Grioni S, Contiero P, Berrino F, Krogh V. Dietary glycemic index, glycemic load, and the risk of breast cancer in an Italian prospective cohort study. *American Journal of Clinical Nutrition.* Oct;86(4):1160-6.

Silvera SA, Jain M, Howe GR, Miller AB, Rohan TE. Dietary carbohydrates and breast cancer risk: a prospective study of the roles of overall glycemic index and glycemic load. *International Journal of Cancer.* 2005 Apr 20;114(4):653-8.

Silvera SA, Rohan TE, Jain M, Terry PD, Howe GR, Miller AB. Glycaemic index, glycaemic load and risk of endometrial cancer: a prospective cohort study. *Public Health Nutrition.* 2005 Oct;8(7):912-9.

CHAPTER 4

American Heart Association. A History of Trans Fat. www.american heart.org/presenter.jhtml?identifier=3048193. Accessed Feb. 6, 2009.

Ban Trans Fats: The Campaign to Ban Partially Hydrogenated Oils. www.bantransfats.com/abouttransfat.html. Accessed Feb. 4, 2009.

Freeman EW, Sammel MD, Grisso JA, Battistini M, Garcia-Espagna B, Hollander L. Hot flashes in the late reproductive years: risk factors for African American and Caucasian women. *Journal of Women's Health & Gender-Based Medicine.* 2001 Jan-Feb;10(1):67-76.

Hui LL, Nelson EA, Choi KC, Wong GW, Sung R. Twelve-hour glycemic profiles with meals of high, medium, or low glycemic load. *Diabetes Care.* 2005 Dec;28(12):2981-3.

Hyde Riley E, Inui TS, Kleinman K, Connelly MT. Differential association of modifiable health behaviors with hot flashes in perimenopausal and postmenopausal women. *Journal of General Internal Medicine.* 2004 July;19(7):740-6.

Ludwig DS. The glycemic index: physiological mechanisms relating to obesity, diabetes, and cardiovascular disease. *Journal of the American Medical Association.* 2002 May 8;287(18):2414-23.

Mozaffarian D. Trans fatty acids–effects on systemic inflammation and endothelial function. *Atherosclerosis. Supplements.* 2006 May; 7(2):29-32. Epub 2006 May 18.

Mozaffarian D, Katan MB, Ascherio A, Stampfer MJ, Willett WC. Trans fatty acids and cardiovascular disease. *New England Journal of Medicine.* 2006 Apr 13;354(15):1601-13.

Mozaffarian D, Willett WC. Trans fatty acids and cardiovascular risk: a unique cardiometabolic imprint? *Current Atherosclerosis Reports.* 2007 Dec;9(6):486-93.

O'Keefe JH, Gheewala NM, O'Keefe JO. Dietary strategies for improving post-prandial glucose, lipids, inflammation, and cardiovascular health. *Journal of the American College of Cardiology.* 2008 Jan 22;51(3):249-55.

Thurston RC, Sowers MR, Sutton-Tyrrell K, Everson-Rose SA, Lewis TT, Edmundowicz D, Matthews KA. Abdominal adiposity and hot flashes among midlife women. *Menopause.* 2008 May-Jun; 15(3):429-34.

Whiteman MK, Staropoli CA, Langenberg PW, McCarter RJ, Kjerulff KH, Flaws JA. Smoking, body mass, and hot flashes in midlife women. *Obstetrics and Gynecology.* 2003 Feb;101(2):264-72.

CHAPTER 5

Bellisle F, Drewnowski A. Intense sweeteners, energy intake and the control of body weight. *European Journal of Clinical Nutrition.* 2007 Jun;61(6):691-700.

Covas MI, Nyyssönen K, Poulsen HE, Kaikkonen J, Zunft HJ, Kiesewetter H, Gaddi A, de la Torre R, Mursu J, Bäumler H, Nascetti S, Salonen JT, Fitó M, Virtanen J, Marrugat J, EUROLIVE Study Group. The effect of polyphenols in olive oil on heart disease risk factors: a randomized trial. *Annals of Internal Medicine.* 2006 Sep 5;145(5):333-41.

Frank GK, Oberndorfer TA, Simmons AN, Paulus MP, Fudge JL, Yang TT, Kaye WH. Sucrose activates human taste pathways differently from artificial sweetener. *Neuroimage.* 2008 Feb 15;39(4): 1559-69.

Halvorsen BL, Carlsen MH, Phillips KM, Bohn SK, Holte K, Jacobs DR Jr, Blomhoff R. Content of redox-active compounds (ie, antioxidants) in foods consumed in the United States. *American Journal of Clinical Nutrition.* 2006 Jul;84(1):95-135.

Hampton T. Sugar substitutes linked to weight gain. *Journal of the American Medical Association.* 2008 May 14;299(18):2137-8.

Jeanelle Boyer J, Hai Liu R. Apple phytochemicals and their health benefits. *Nutrition Journal.* 2004 May 12;3:5.

Lucas EA, Wild RD, Hammond LJ, Khalil DA, Juma S, Daggy BP, Stoecker BJ, Arjmandi BH. Flaxseed improves lipid profile without altering biomarkers of bone metabolism in postmenopausal women. *The Journal of Clinical Endocrinology and Metabolism.* 2002 Apr;87(4):1527-32.

O'Keefe JH, Gheewala NM, O'Keefe JO. Dietary strategies for

improving post-prandial glucose, lipids, inflammation, and cardio-vascular health. *Journal of the American College of Cardiology.* 2008 Jan 22;51(3):249-55.

Ostman E, Granfeldt Y, Persson L, Björck I. Vinegar supplementation lowers glucose and insulin responses and increases satiety after a bread meal in healthy subjects. *European Journal of Clinical Nutrition.* 2005 Sep;59(9):983-8.

Salas-Salvadó J, Fernández-Ballart J, Ros E, Martínez-González MA, Fitó M, Estruch R, Corella D, Fiol M, Gómez-Gracia E, Arós F, Flores G, Lapetra J, Lamuela-Raventós R, Ruiz-Gutiérrez V, Bulló M, Basora J, Covas MI, PREDIMED Study Investigators. Effect of a Mediterranean diet supplemented with nuts on metabolic syndrome status: one-year results of the PREDIMED randomized trial. *Archives of Internal Medicine.* 2008 Dec 8;168(22):2449-58.

Surette ME. The science behind dietary omega-3 fatty acids. *Canadian Medical Association Journal.* 2008 Jan 15;178(2):177-80.

World Cancer Research Fund and American Institute for Cancer Research. *Food, Nutrition, Physical Activity, and the Prevention of Cancer: a Global Perspective.* Washington DC: AICR, 2007.

CHAPTER 6

Curtis BM, O'Keefe JH Jr. Autonomic tone as a cardiovascular risk factor: the dangers of chronic fight or flight. *Mayo Clinic Proceedings.* 2002;77:45-54.

Durrant-Peatfield B. *Your Thyroid and How To Keep It Healthy.* London, UK: Hammersmith Press Limited, 2008.

Fowler JH, Christakis NA. Dynamic spread of happiness in a large social network: longitudinal analysis over 20 years in the Framingham Heart Study. *British Medical Journal.* 2008 Dec 4;337: a2338.

McEwen BS, Sapolsky RM. Stress and cognitive function. *Current Opinion in Neurobiology.* 1995 Apr;5(2):205-16.

Sapolsky RM. *Why Zebras Don't Get Ulcers.* New York, NY: Holt Paperbacks, 2004.

Segar M, Jayaratne T, Hanlon J, Richardson CR. Fitting fitness into women's lives: effects of a gender-tailored physical activity inter-vention. *Womens Health Issues.* 2002 Nov-Dec;12(6):338-47.

Segar ML, Eccles JS, Richardson CR. Type of physical activity goal influences participation in healthy midlife women. *Womens Health Issues.* 2008 Jul-Aug;18(4):281-91.

Teitelbaum J. *From Fatigued to Fantastic.* New York, NY: Avery, 2007.

Wilson JL. *Adrenal Fatigue.* Petaluma, CA: Smart Publications, 2007.

Woods NF, Carr MC, Tao EY, Taylor HJ, Mitchell ES. Increased urinary cortisol levels during the menopausal transition. *Menopause.* 2006 Mar-Apr;13(2):212-21.

CHAPTER 7

Crain DA, Janssen SJ, Edwards TM, Heindel J, Ho SM, Hunt P, Iguchi T, Juul A, McLachlan JA, Schwartz J, Skakkebaek N, Soto AM, Swan S, Walker C, Woodruff TK, Woodruff TJ, Giudice LC, Guillette LJ Jr. Female reproductive disorders: the roles of endocrine-disrupting compounds and developmental timing. *Fertility and Sterility.* 2008 Oct;90(4):911-40.

Environmental Working Group. *Shopper's Guide to Pesticides.* www.foodnews.org.

Institute for Children's Environmental Health. Plastics: A Fact Sheet. www.iceh.org/pdfs/SBLF/PlasticsFactSheet.pdf. Accessed March 2, 2009.

Lu C, Toepel K, Irish R, Fenske RA, Barr DB, Bravo R. Organic diets significantly lower children's dietary exposure to organophosphorus pesticides. *Environmental Health Perspectives.* 2006 Feb;114(2):260-3.

McCullum-Gomez C, Benbrook C, Theuer R. *Critical Issue Report: That First Step–Organic Food and a Healthier Future.* The Organic Center. March 2009. www.organic-center.org.

National Institute of Environmental Health Sciences–National Institutes of Health. *Endocrine Disruptors.* http://www.niehs.nih.gov/health/topics/agents/endocrine/docs/endocrine.pdf. Accessed April 5, 2009.

Pennybacker, M. *Antibacterials? Here's the Rub.* Worldwatch Institute. www.worldwatch.org/system/files/GS0025.pdf. Accessed March 2, 2009.

Runestad T. Organics: Does the Science Validate It? *Functional Foods & Nutraceuticals.* May 2007;34-42.

United States Department of Agriculture, Agricultural Marketing Service. National Organic Program. www.ams.usda.gov/nop.

Veldhoen N, Skirrow RC, Osachoff H, Wigmore H, Clapson DJ,

Gunderson MP, Van Aggelen G, Helbing CC. The bactericidal agent triclosan modulates thyroid hormone-associated gene expression and disrupts postembryonic anuran development. *Aquatic Toxicology*. 2006 Dec 1;80(3):217-27.

Women's Reproductive Health and the Environment Workshop at Commonweal, Bolinas, CA, January 6–9, 2008. *Hormone Disruptors and Women's Health: Reasons for Concern.* Accessed from www.womenshealthandenvironment.org March 2, 2009.

CHAPTER 8

Annesi JJ, Westcott WL. Relations of physical self-concept and muscular strength with resistance exercise-induced feeling state scores in older women. *Perceptual and Motor Skills*. 2007 Feb;104(1):183-90.

Annesi JJ, Westcott WL. Relationship of feeling states after exercise and total mood disturbance over 10 weeks in formerly sedentary women. *Perceptual and Motor Skills*. 2004 Aug;99(1):107-15.

Boulé NG, Haddad E, Kenny GP, Wells GA, Sigal RJ. Effects of exercise on glycemic control and body mass in Type 2 diabetes mellitus: a meta-analysis of controlled clinical trials. *Journal of the American Medical Association*. 2001 Sep 12;286(10):1218-27.

Martins C, Morgan LM, Bloom SR, Robertson MD. Effects of exercise on gut peptides, energy intake and appetite. *The Journal of Endocrinology*. 2007 May;193(2):251-8.

Martins C, Robertson MD, Morgan LM. Effects of exercise and restrained eating behaviour on appetite control. *The Proceedings of the Nutrition Society*. 2008 Feb;67(1):28-41.

Schmaltz J, Lehrhoff S, Anderson P (Eds). *The Healing Power of Exercise.* International Health, Racquet & Sportsclub Association, 2008.

Shephard RJ. Maximal oxygen intake and independence in old age. *British Journal of Sports Medicine*. 2008 Apr 10. [Epub ahead of print].

Vella CA, Kravitz L. Sarcopenia: The mystery of muscle loss. *IDEA Personal Trainer*. 2002;13(4):30-5.

Westcott WL, Winett RA. Applying the ACSM Guidelines. *Fitness Management*. January 2006.

Williams PT. Prospective epidemiological cohort study of reduced risk for incident cataract with vigorous physical activity and cardiorespiratory fitness during a 7-year follow-up. *Investigative*

Ophthalmology and Visual Science. 2009 Jan;50(1):95-100.

Williams PT. Prospective study of incident age-related macular degeneration in relation to vigorous physical activity during a 7-year follow-up. *Investigative Ophthalmology and Visual Science.* 2009 Jan;50(1):101-6.

CHAPTER 9

Balch P, Balch J. *Prescription for Nutritional Healing.* New York, NY: Avery, 2000.

Christen WG, Glynn RJ, Chew EY, Albert CM, Manson JE. Folic acid, pyridoxine, and cyanocobalamin combination treatment and age-related macular degeneration in women: the Women's Antioxidant and Folic Acid Cardiovascular Study. *Archives of Internal Medicine.* 2009 Feb 23;169(4):335-41.

Dowd JE, Stafford D. *The Vitamin D Cure.* Hoboken, NJ: Wiley, 2009.

Grimm T, Chovanová Z, Muchová J, Sumegová K, Liptáková A, Duracková Z, Högger P. Inhibition of NF-kappaB activation and MMP-9 secretion by plasma of human volunteers after ingestion of maritime pine bark extract (Pycnogenol). *Journal of inflammation (London, England).* 2006 Jan 27;3:1.

Hu Y, Block G, Norkus EP, Morrow JD, Dietrich M, Hudes M. Relations of glycemic index and glycemic load with plasma oxidative stress markers. *American Journal of Clinical Nutrition.* 2006 Jul;84(1):70-6.

Keaney JF Jr, Larson MG, Vasan RS, Wilson PW, Lipinska I, Corey D, Massaro JM, Sutherland P, Vita JA, Benjamin EJ; Framingham Study. Obesity and systemic oxidative stress: clinical correlates of oxidative stress in the Framingham Study. *Arteriosclerosis, Thrombosis, and Vascular Biology.* 2003 Mar 1;23(3):434-9.

Langsjoen PH, Langsjoen AM. Overview of the use of CoQ10 in cardiovascular disease. *Biofactors.* 1999;9(2-4):273-84.

Lucas M, Asselin G, Mérette C, Poulin MJ, Dodin S. Effects of ethyl-eicosapentaenoic acid omega-3 fatty acid supplementation on hot flashes and quality of life among middle-aged women: a double-blind, placebo-controlled, randomized clinical trial. *Menopause.* 2009 March/April;16(2):357-66.

Lucas M, Asselin G, Mérette C, Poulin MJ, Dodin S. Ethyl-eicosapentaenoic acid for the treatment of psychological distress and depressive symptoms in middle-aged women: a double-blind, placebo-controlled, randomized clinical trial. *American Journal of Clinical Nutrition.* 2009 Feb;89(2):641-51.

Matthews RT, Yang L, Browne S, Baik M, Beal MF. Coenzyme Q10 administration increases brain mitochondrial concentrations and exerts neuroprotective effects. *Proceedings of the National Academy of Sciences of the United States of America.* 1998 Jul 21;95(15):8892-7.

Moore CE, Murphy MM, Holick MF. Vitamin D intakes by children and adults in the United States differ among ethnic groups. *Journal of Nutrition.* 2005 Oct;135(10):2478-85.

Morisco C, Trimarco B, Condorelli M. Effect of coenzyme Q10 therapy in patients with congestive heart failure: a long-term multicenter randomized study. *The Clinical Investigator.* 1993;71(8 Suppl): S134-6.

Seelig M. *The Magnesium Factor.* New York, NY: Avery, 2003.

Singh RB, Wander GS, Rastogi A, et al. Randomized, double-blind placebo-controlled trial of coenzyme Q10 in patients with acute myocardial infarction. *Cardiovascular Drugs and Therapy.* 1998; 12(4):347-53.

Tarpila S, Aro A, Salminen I, Tarpila A, Kleemola P, Akkila J, Adlercreutz H. The effect of flaxseed supplementation in processed foods on serum fatty acids and enterolactone. *European Journal of Clinical Nutrition.* 2002 Feb;56(2):157-65.

Thompson HJ, Heimendinger J, Sedlacek S, Haegele A, Diker A, O'Neill C, Meinecke B, Wolfe P, Zhu Z, Jiang W. 8-Isoprostane F2alpha excretion is reduced in women by increased vegetable and fruit intake. *American Journal of Clinical Nutrition.* 2005 Oct;82(4): 768-76.

CHAPTER 10

Aggarwal BB, Ichikawa H. Molecular targets and anticancer potential of indole-3-carbinol and its derivatives. *Cell Cycle.* 2005 Sep;4(9): 1201-15.

Arthritis Foundation. What being overweight does to your OA risk. www.arthritistoday.org/conditions/osteoarthritis/news-and-research/osteoarthritis-weight.php. Accessed April 8, 2009.

Bissessar EA, Watkins PJ, Sampson M, et al. Treatment of diabetic neuropathy with gamma-linolenic acid. The gamma-linolenic acid multicenter trial group. *Diabetes Care.* 1993 Jan;16(1):8-15.

Bohager T. *Enzymes: What The Experts Know*. Prescott, AZ: One World Press, 2006.

Cangiano C, Ceci F, Cascino A, Del Ben M, Laviano A, Muscaritoli M, Antonucci F, Rossi-Fanelli F. Eating behavior and adherence to dietary prescriptions in obese adult subjects treated with 5-hydroxytryptophan. *American Journal of Clinical Nutrition*. 1992 Nov; 56(5):863-7.

Cutler EW, Kaslow JE. *Micro Miracles: Discover the Healing Power of Enzymes*. Emmaus, PA: Rodale Books, 2005.

Goldin BR, Gorbach SL. Clinical indications for probiotics: an overview. *Clinical Infectious Diseases*. 2008 Feb 1;46 Suppl 2:S96-100.

Haskell CF, Kennedy DO, Milne AL, Wesnes KA, Scholey AB. The effects of L-theanine, caffeine and their combination on cognition and mood. *Biological Psychology*. 2008 Feb;77(2):113-22.

Horrobin DF. Evening primrose oil and premenstrual syndrome. *The Medical Journal of Australia*. 1990 Nov 19;153(10):630-1.

Horrobin DF. Nutritional and medical importance of gamma-linolenic acid. *Progress in Lipid Research*. 1992;31(2):163-94.

Jepson RG, Craig JC. A systematic review of the evidence for cranberries and blueberries in UTI prevention. *Molecular Nutrition & Food Research*. 2007 Jun;51(6):738-45.

Keen H, Payan J, Allawi J, Walker J, Jamal GA, Weir AI, Henderson LM, Kimura K, Ozeki M, Juneja LR, Ohira H. L-Theanine reduces psychological and physiological stress responses. *Biological Psychology*. 2007 Jan;74(1):39-45.

Kligler B, Cohrssen A. Probiotics. *American Family Physician*. 2008 Nov 1;78(9):1073-8.

Leonhardt M, Langhans W. Fatty acid oxidation and control of food intake. *Physiology and Behavior*. 2004 83(4):645-51.

Li Y, Li X, Sarkar FH. Gene expression profiles of I3C- and DIM-treated PC3 human prostate cancer cells determined by cDNA microarray analysis. *The Journal of Nutrition*. 2003 Apr;133(4):1011-9.

McMurdo ME, Argo I, Phillips G, Daly F, Davey P. Cranberry or trimethoprim for the prevention of recurrent urinary tract infections? A randomized controlled trial in older women. *Journal of Antimicrobial Chemotherapy*. 2009 Feb;63(2):389-95.

Nappi RE, Malavasi B, Brundu B, Facchinetti F. Efficacy of Cimicifuga racemosa on climacteric complaints: a randomized study versus low-dose transdermal estradiol. *Gynecological Endocrinology.* 2005 Jan;20(1):30-5.

Office of Dietary Supplements, National Institutes of Health. Carnitine. http://dietary-supplements.info.nih.gov/factsheets/carnitine.asp.

Osmers R, Friede M, Liske E, Schnitker J, Freudenstein J, Henneicke-von Zepelin HH. Efficacy and safety of isopropanolic black cohosh extract for climacteric symptoms. *Obstetrics and Gynecology.* 2005 May;105(5 Pt 1):1074-83.

Prasad K. Dietary flax seed in prevention of hypercholesterolemic atherosclerosis. *Atherosclerosis.* 1997 Jul 11;132(1):69-76.

Preuss H, Gottlieb B. *The Natural Fat-Loss Pharmacy.* New York, NY: Broadway Books, 2007.

Rahman KM, Aranha O, Sarkar FH. Indole-3-carbinol (I3C) induces apoptosis in tumorigenic but not in nontumorigenic breast epithelial cells. *Nutrition and Cancer.* 2003;45(1):101-12.

Tarpila S, Kivinen A. Ground flaxseed is an effective hypolipidemic bulk laxative [abstract]. *Gastroenterology.* 1997 112:A836.

CHAPTER II

Breslau ES, Davis WW, Doner L, Eisner EJ, Goodman NR, Meissner HI, Rimer BK, Rossouw JE. The hormone therapy dilemma: women respond. *Journal of the American Medical Women's Association.* 2003 Winter;58(1):33-43.

Chlebowski RT, Kuller LH, Prentice RL, Stefanick ML, Manson JE, Gass M, Aragaki AK, Ockene JK, Lane DS, Sarto GE, Rajkovic A, Schenken R, Hendrix SL, Ravdin PM, Rohan TE, Yasmeen S, Anderson G; WHI Investigators. Breast cancer after use of estrogen plus progestin in postmenopausal women. *New England Journal of Medicine.* 2009 Feb 5;360(6):573-87.

Fitzpatrick LA, Pace C, Wiita B. Comparison of regimens containing oral micronized progesterone or medroxyprogesterone acetate on quality of life in postmenopausal women: a cross-sectional survey. *Journal of Women's Health & Gender-Based Medicine.* 2000 May; 9(4):381-7.

Fournier A, Berrino F, Clavel-Chapelon F. Unequal risks for breast cancer associated with different hormone replacement therapies: results from the E3N cohort study. *Breast Cancer Research and Treatment.* 2008 Jan;107(1):103-11.

Fournier A, Berrino F, Riboli E, Avenel V, Clavel-Chapelon F. Breast cancer risk in relation to different types of hormone replacement therapy in the E3N-EPIC cohort. *International Journal of Cancer.* 2005 Apr 10;114(3):448-54.

Holtorf K. The bioidentical hormone debate: are bioidentical hormones (estradiol, estriol, and progesterone) safer or more efficacious than commonly used synthetic versions in hormone replacement therapy? *Postgraduate Medicine.* 2009 Jan;121(1):73-85.

Manson JE, Hsia J, Johnson KC, Rossouw JE, Assaf AR, Lasser NL, Trevisan M, Black HR, Heckbert SR, Detrano R, Strickland OL, Wong ND, Crouse JR, Stein E, Cushman M; Women's Health Initiative Investigators. Estrogen plus progestin and the risk of coronary heart disease. *New England Journal of Medicine.* 2003 Aug 7;349(6):523-34.

Power ML, Schulkin J, Rossouw JE. Evolving practice patterns and attitudes toward hormone therapy of obstetrician-gynecologists. *Menopause.* 2007 Jan-Feb;14(1):20-8.

Rossouw JE. Implications of recent clinical trials of postmenopausal hormone therapy for management of cardiovascular disease. *Annals of the New York Academy of Sciences.* 2006 Nov;1089:444-53.

Rossouw JE, Anderson GL, Prentice RL, LaCroix AZ, Kooperberg C, Stefanick ML, Jackson RD, Beresford SA, Howard BV, Johnson KC, Kotchen JM, Ockene J; Writing Group for the Women's Health Initiative Investigators. Risks and benefits of estrogen plus progestin in healthy postmenopausal women: principal results from the Women's Health Initiative randomized controlled trial. *Journal of the American Medical Association.* 2002 Jul 17;288(3):321-33.

Rossouw JE, Cushman M, Greenland P, Lloyd-Jones DM, Bray P, Kooperberg C, Pettinger M, Robinson J, Hendrix S, Hsia J. Inflammatory, lipid, thrombotic, and genetic markers of coronary heart disease risk in the women's health initiative trials of hormone therapy. *Archives of Internal Medicine.* 2008 Nov 10;168(20):2245-53.

Rossouw JE, Prentice RL, Manson JE, Wu L, Barad D, Barnabei VM, Ko M, LaCroix AZ, Margolis KL, Stefanick ML. Postmenopausal hormone therapy and risk of cardiovascular disease by age and years since menopause. *Journal of the American Medical Association.* 2007 Apr 4;297(13):1465-77.

Schwartz ET, Holtorf K. Hormones in wellness and disease prevention: common practices, current state of the evidence, and questions for the future. *Primary Care*. 2008 Dec;35(4):669-705.

Stephenson K, Kurdowska A, Neuenschwander P, Loewenstein I, Olusola P, Pinson B, Stephenson D, Kinsey R, Stephenson J, Kapur S, Zava D. Transdermal estradiol and progesterone improve mood indicators, quality of life, and biomarkers of cardiovascular disease in perimenopausal and postmenopausal women. *Circulation*. 2007 Feb 27;115(8):e277.

Wassertheil-Smoller S, Hendrix SL, Limacher M, Heiss G, Kooperberg C, Baird A, Kotchen T, Curb JD, Black H, Rossouw JE, Aragaki A, Safford M, Stein E, Laowattana S, Mysiw WJ; WHI Investigators. Effect of estrogen plus progestin on stroke in postmenopausal women: the Women's Health Initiative: a randomized trial. *Journal of the American Medical Association*. 2003 May 28; 289(20):2673-84.

CHAPTER 12

Ahlgrimm M. Managing PMS and perimenopause symptoms. The role of compounded medications. *Advance for Nurse Practitioners*. 2003 May;11(5):53-4, 90.

Barnes BO, Galton L. *Hypothyroidism: The Unsuspected Illness*. New York, NY: HarperCollins, 1976.

Durrant-Peatfield B. *Your Thyroid and How to Keep Healthy*. London, UK: Hammersmith Press Ltd, 2006.

Edelman A, Stouffer R, Zava DT, Jensen JT. A comparison of blood spot vs. plasma analysis of gonadotropin and ovarian steroid hormone levels in reproductive-age women. *Fertility and Sterility*. 2007 Nov;88(5):1404-7.

Ghen MJ, Russell SL. *Anti-Aging Physicians' Handbook for Compounding Pharmaceuticals*. Birmingham, AL: Ghen/Russell, 2008.

Glaser RL, Zava DT, Wurtzbacher D. Pilot study: absorption and efficacy of multiple hormones delivered in a single cream applied to the mucous membranes of the labia and vagina. *Gynecologic and Obstetric Investigation*. 2008;66(2):111-8.

International Academy of Compounding Pharmacists. www.iacprx.org.

Kronenberg HM, Melmed S, Polonsky KS, Reed Larsen (Eds). *Williams Textbook of Endocrinology*. Philadelphia, PA: Saunders, 2007.

Laughlin GA, Barrett-Connor E, Bergstrom J. Low serum testosterone and mortality in older men. *The Journal of Clinical Endocrinology and Metabolism.* 2008 Jan;93(1):68-75.

Moskowitz D. A comprehensive review of the safety and efficacy of bioidentical hormones for the management of menopause and related health risks. *Alternative Medicine Review.* 2006;11(3):208-23.

Smith PW. *HRT: The Answers.* Traverse City, MI: Healthy Living Books, 2003.

William Mck J. *Safe Uses of Cortisol.* Springfield, IL: Charles C Thomas Publisher Ltd, 2004.

CHAPTER 13

American College of Sports Medicine. *ACSM's Guidelines for Exercise Testing and Prescription.* Philadelphia, PA: Lippincott Williams & Wilkins, 2009.

American Dietetic Association. Nutrition and You: Trends 2008. www.eatright.org/trends2008. Accessed March 23, 2009.

American Heart Association. *Heart Disease and Stroke Statistics–2009 Update.* Dallas, Texas: American Heart Association; 2009.

Baillie-Hamilton P. *Toxic Overload.* New York, NY: Avery, 2005.

Brand-Miller J. Effects of glycemic load on weight loss in overweight adults. *American Journal of Clinical Nutrition.* 2007 Oct;86(4): 1249-50.

Food and Nutrition Board, Institute of Medicine. *Dietary Reference Intakes for Energy, Carbohydrate, Fiber, Fat, Fatty Acids, Cholesterol, Protein, and Amino Acids (Macronutrients).* Washington, DC: The National Academies Press, 2005.

McMillan-Price J, Petocz P, Atkinson F, O'Neill K, Samman S, Steinbeck K, Caterson I, Brand-Miller J. Comparison of 4 diets of varying glycemic load on weight loss and cardiovascular risk reduction in overweight and obese young adults: a randomized controlled trial. *Archives of Internal Medicine.* 2006 Jul 24;166(14):1466-75.

Simin L. Lowering dietary glycemic load for weight control and cardiovascular health. *Archives of Internal Medicine.* 2006 Jul 24;166(14): 1438-9.

World Cancer Research Fund/American Institute for Cancer Research. *Food, Nutrition, Physical Activity, and the Prevention of Cancer: a Global Perspective.* Washington DC: AICR, 2007.

Wyatt HR, Grunwald GK, Mosca CL, Klem ML, Wing RR, Hill JO.

Long-term weight loss and breakfast in subjects in the National Weight Control Registry. *Obesity Research.* 2002 Feb;10(2):78-82.

CHAPTER 14

Almeida OP, Yeap BB, Hankey GJ, Jamrozik K, Flicker L. Low free testosterone concentration as a potentially treatable cause of depressive symptoms in older men. *Archives of General Psychiatry.* 2008 Mar;65(3):283-9.

Chavarro JE, Stampfer MJ, Hall MN, Sesso HD, Ma J. A 22-y prospective study of fish intake in relation to prostate cancer incidence and mortality. *American Journal of Clinical Nutrition.* 2008 Nov;88(5):1297-303.

Debruyne F, Koch G, Boyle P, Da Silva FC, Gillenwater JG, Hamdy FC, Perrin P, Teillac P, Vela-Navarrete R, Raynaud JP. Comparison of a phytotherapeutic agent (Permixon) with an alpha-blocker (Tamsulosin) in the treatment of benign prostatic hyperplasia: a 1-year randomized international study. *European Urology.* 2002 May;41(5):497-506.

Gerber GS, Kuznetsov D, Johnson BC, Burstein JD. Randomized, double-blind, placebo-controlled trial of saw palmetto in men with lower urinary tract symptoms. *Urology.* 2001 Dec;58(6):960-4.

Hall SA, Esche GR, Araujo AB, Travison TG, Clark RV, Williams RE, McKinlay JB. Correlates of low testosterone and symptomatic androgen deficiency in a population-based sample. *The Journal of Clinical Endocrinology and Metabolism.* 2008 Oct;93(10):3870-7.

Hall SA, Kupelian V, Rosen RC, Travison TG, Link CL, Miner MM, Ganz P, McKinlay JB. Is hyperlipidemia or its treatment associated with erectile dysfunction?: Results from the Boston Area Community Health (BACH) Survey. *The Journal of Sexual Medicine.* 2009 May;6(5):1402-13.

Hsing AW, Gao YT, Chua S Jr, Deng J, Stanczyk FZ. Insulin resistance and prostate cancer risk. *Journal of the National Cancer Institute.* 2003 Jan 1;95(1):67-71.

Moffat SD, Zonderman AB, Metter EJ, Kawas C, Blackman MR, Harman SM, Resnick SM. Free testosterone and risk for Alzheimer's disease in older men. *Neurology.* 2004 Jan 27;62(2):188-93.

Muller M, van der Schouw YT, Thijssen JH, Grobbee DE. Endogenous sex hormones and cardiovascular disease in men. *The Journal of*

Clinical Endocrinology and Metabolism. 2003 Nov;88(11):5076-86.

Rhoden EL, Morgentaler A. Risks of testosterone-replacement therapy and recommendations for monitoring. *New England Journal of Medicine.* 2004 Jan 29;350(5):482-92.

Stattin P, Lumme S, Tenkanen L, Alfthan H, Jellum E, Hallmans G, Thoresen S, Hakulinen T, Luostarinen T, Lehtinen M, Dillner J, Stenman UH, Hakama M. High levels of circulating testosterone are not associated with increased prostate cancer risk: a pooled prospective study. *International Journal of Cancer.* 2004 Jan 20;108(3):418-24.

Swan SH. Environmental phthalate exposure in relation to reproductive outcomes and other health endpoints in humans. *Environmental Research.* 2008 Oct;108(2):177-84.

Travison TG, Araujo AB, Kupelian V, O'Donnell AB, McKinlay JB. The relative contributions of aging, health, and lifestyle factors to serum testosterone decline in men. *The Journal of Clinical Endocrinology and Metabolism.* 2007 Feb;92(2):549-55.

Travison TG, Araujo AB, O'Donnell AB, Kupelian V, McKinlay JB. A population-level decline in serum testosterone levels in American men. *The Journal of Clinical Endocrinology and Metabolism.* 2007 Jan;92(1):196-202.

Travison TG, Shabsigh R, Araujo AB, Kupelian V, O'Donnell AB, McKinlay JB. The natural progression and remission of erectile dysfunction: results from the Massachusetts Male Aging Study. *Journal of Urology.* 2007 Jan;177(1):241-6.

INDEX

I3C (Indole-3 Carbinol) and, 131
enzymes, 112, 114
  digestive, 127-128, 131
EPA (eicosapentaenoic acid), 116-118
erectile dysfunction, 174, 178
estrogen
  aging and, 5-6
  bioidentical, use of, 143, 153, 155, 191
  black cohosh and, 124
  cancer and, 9, 131, 141
  conversion, in men, 180
  dominance, 19
  HRT and, 137-138
  insulin and, 14
  role of, 150
  synthetic, 137
  tests, 151-152
  toxins and, 75, 82
exercise
  aerobic, 92-97, 99
  important reasons to, 90-91
  strength training, 88-93, 97, 99-102
  to reduce stress, 68-74

fast food, 13, 21-23, 41, 47, 167, 175
fat cells, 16, 17, 181
fatigue, chronic, 106, 129
fats, dietary
  healthy, 38, 50-51, 56, 125, 162
  saturated, 13, 16, 38-39, 53, 182
  trans, 16, 38-44, 52
fish oil, benefits of, 115-117, 119, 121
5-HTP, 126-127, 131
flaxseed, 38, 51, 130
  oil, 44, 51, 115, 118, 121
folic acid, 108-109, 120
food
  additives, 75, 80, 185
  cravings, 54, 162
  labels, 31, 39-40, 42, 44, 53, 78-80
  low-fat, 12-13, 164

organic, benefits, 76-80, 85, 167, 171, 185
plant, 105-106, 112, 115, 118
processed, 12, 38, 41, 43, 47, 53, 125, 164
sensitivities, 59
timing, 37
fragrance, 82-86, 167, 171, 185

GLA (gamma-linolenic acid), 125
gluten, 58
glycemic index (GI), 27-32
grape seed extract, 106-107

heart rate, 94-97
  monitor, 95-97
herbal tea, 29, 44, 57, 163, 170
herbs, as medicine, 126, 148, 186
high fructose corn syrup. *See* sweeteners
hormonal malfunction, 4-6, 14-20, 114, 152
  in men, 179, 183-184
hormones, why tested, 142-143, 145-146, 149, 151-152
  costs of tests, 157-158
Hormone Harmony Habits Checklist, 170-171
hormone replacement therapy (HRT), 8-9, 133, 137-143
hot flashes
  triggers of, 3, 19, 34
  exercise and, 97
  remedies for, 111, 115, 123-127, 135
  bioidentical hormones and, 133, 135, 141, 143, 145, 151
  HRT and, 138

incontinence, and exercise, 91
indole-3-carbinol (I3C), 131
insulin
  age-related increase, 6
  chromium and, 113
  cortisol and, 17